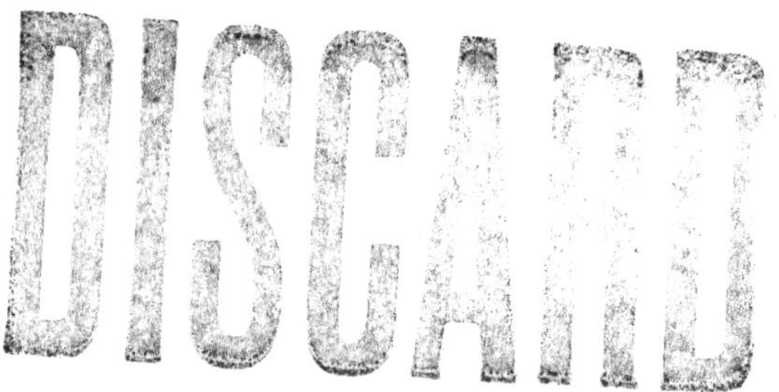

NUTRITION & HEALTH

Sleep Problems

TITLES IN THIS SERIES INCLUDE:

Childhood Obesity

Diet and Disease

Eating Disorders

Food Allergies

Food Myths and Facts

Food Regulation and Safety

Genetically Modified Foods

Junk Food Junkies

Vaccines

Vegetarianism

NUTRITION & HEALTH

Sleep Problems

DON NARDO

LUCENT BOOKS
A part of Gale, Cengage Learning

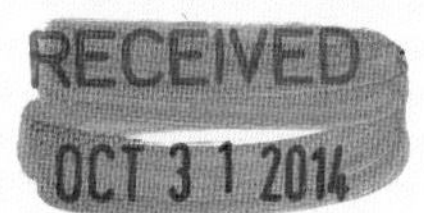

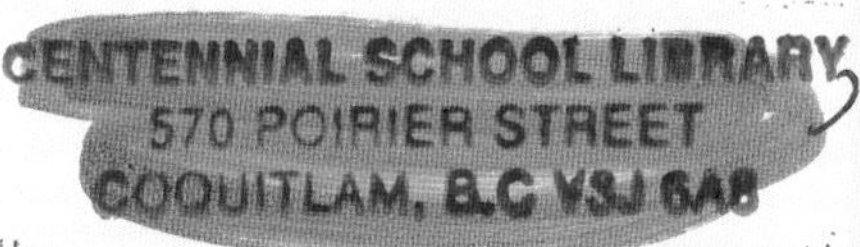

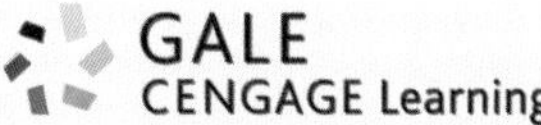

Detroit • New York • San Francisco • New Haven, Conn • Waterville, Maine • London

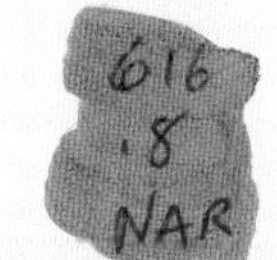

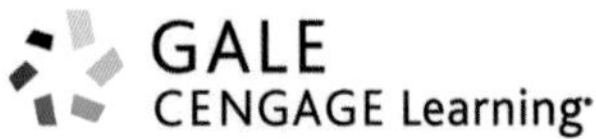

LIBRARY OF CONGRESS CATALOGING-IN-PUBLICATION DATA

Nardo, Don, 1947-
Sleep problems / by Don Nardo.
pages cm -- (Nutrition and health)
Includes bibliographical references and index.
ISBN 978-1-4205-1150-5 (hardcover)
1. Sleep disorders. 2. Sleep disorders--Treatment. 3. Diet therapy.
4. Self-care, Health. I. Title.
RC547.N37 2014
616.8'498--dc23

2013028314

Lucent Books
27500 Drake Rd.
Farmington Hills, MI 48331

ISBN-13: 978-1-4205-1150-5
ISBN-10: 1-4205-1150-5

Printed in the United States of America
1 2 3 4 5 6 7 17 16 15 14 13

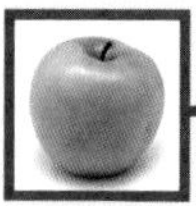

TABLE OF CONTENTS

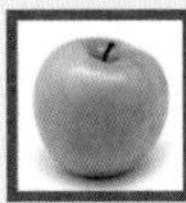

FOREWORD

Many people today are often amazed by the amount of nutrition and health information, often contradictory, that can be found in the media. Television, newspapers, and magazines bombard readers with the latest news and recommendations. Television news programs report on recent scientific studies. The healthy living sections of newspapers and magazines offer information and advice. In addition, electronic media such as websites, blogs, and forums post daily nutrition and health news and recommendations.

This constant stream of information can be confusing. The science behind nutrition and health is constantly evolving. Current research often leads to new ideas and insights. Many times, the latest nutrition studies and health recommendations contradict previous studies or traditional health advice. When the media reports these changes without giving context or explanations, consumers become confused. In a survey by the National Health Council, for example, 68 percent of participants agreed that "when reporting medical and health news, the media often contradict themselves, so I don't know what to believe." In addition, the Food Marketing Institute reported that eight out of ten consumers thought it was likely that nutrition and health experts would have a completely different idea about what foods are healthy within five years. With so much contradictory information, people have difficulty deciding how to apply nutrition and health recommendations to their lives. Students find it difficult to find relevant, yet clear and credible information for reports.

Changing recommendations for antioxidant supplements are an example of how confusion can arise. In the 1990s antioxidants such as vitamins C and E and beta-carotene came to the public's attention. Scientists found that people who ate more antioxidant-rich foods had a lower risk of heart disease, cancer, vision loss, and other chronic conditions than those who ate lower amounts. Without waiting for more scientific study, the media and supplement companies quickly spread the word that antioxidants could help fight and prevent disease. They recommended that people take antioxidant supplements and eat fortified foods. When further scientific studies were completed, however, most did not support the initial recommendations. While naturally occurring antioxidants in fruits and vegetables may help prevent a variety of chronic diseases, little scientific evidence proved antioxidant supplements had the same effect. In fact, a study published in the November 2008 *Journal of the American Medical Association* found that supplemental vitamins A and C gave no more heart protection than a placebo. The study's results contradicted the widely publicized recommendation, leading to consumer confusion. This example highlights the importance of context for evaluating nutrition and health news. Understanding a topic's scientific background, interpreting a study's findings, and evaluating news sources are critical skills that help reduce confusion.

Lucent's Nutrition and Health series is designed to help young people sift through the mountain of confusing facts, opinions, and recommendations. Each book contains the most recent up-to-date information, synthesized and written so that students can understand and think critically about nutrition and health issues. Each volume of the series provides a balanced overview of today's hot-button nutrition and health issues while presenting the latest scientific findings and a discussion of issues surrounding the topic. The series provides young people with tools for evaluating conflicting and ever-changing ideas about nutrition and health. Clear narrative peppered with personal anecdotes, fully documented primary and secondary source quotes, informative sidebars, fact boxes, and statistics are all used to help readers understand these topics and how they affect their bodies and their lives. Each volume includes information about changes in trends over time, political controversies, and international perspectives. Full-color photographs and charts enhance all volumes in the series. The Nutrition and Health series is a valuable resource for young people to understand current topics and make informed choices for themselves.

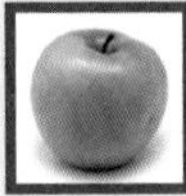

INTRODUCTION

Dispelling a Famous Sleep Myth

There have been many myths perpetuated about sleep over the years. One of them claims that everyone requires eight hours of sleep to function normally. (In reality, sleep requirements vary slightly from person to person, so some people need a little less than eight hours and others a little more.) Another familiar sleep myth, one frequently perpetuated by teachers and parents, suggests that teenagers who are drowsy during their early morning classes lack the discipline to go to bed early. (The truth is that, because they are still growing, teenagers require considerably more sleep than adults and may well be tired in the early morning hours even when they do go to bed early.)

No less often repeated and believed is the sleep myth that claims that many of the world's brilliant, great, or important people need and get far less sleep than "ordinary" humans. Supposedly, these "short sleepers" hate the very idea of having to sleep, because it robs them of precious hours in which they could be creating, inventing, or otherwise helping humanity to progress. One of these notorious sleep haters, the famous American inventor Thomas Edison, said that sleeping through the night was "unhealthy and inefficient." Someone "who sleeps eight or ten hours a night," he stated, "is never fully asleep and never fully awake. They have only different degrees of doze through the twenty-four hours."[1]

Edison claimed he got by on only three or four hours of sleep per night and that he sometimes worked on his inventions for seventy-two hours straight without sleeping at all. Other supposed sleep haters include the Renaissance artist Leonardo da Vinci, the French military general Napoléon Bonaparte, and U.S. founding fathers Benjamin Franklin and Thomas Jefferson. These individuals were said to have slept a little—maybe fifteen to twenty minutes—every four or five hours. Altogether, the story goes, they managed to function perfectly well on a total of two, three, or four hours of sleep a day. Modern sleep experts call this habit of taking periodic tiny naps throughout the day, rather than getting one longer chunk of sleep at night, polyphasic sleeping.

Very Hard to Confirm

The problem with these historical tales of polyphasic sleepers is that closer inspection of their lives does not support the claim that they slept less than other people. Edison is a typical example. It is true that he slept very little during the night. However, it turns out that he took two or three long naps—of two or more hours each—during the daytime and hid the practice from most people.

This fact came to light when the renowned car manufacturer Henry Ford visited Edison's lab one day and asked to see the boss. Edison's chief assistant, who was one of the few people who knew about the inventor's napping habits, told Ford he would have to wait. Edison was asleep on his workbench, the assistant explained, and did not want to be disturbed. "But I thought Edison didn't sleep very much,"[2] Ford responded. With a smile, the assistant said, "He doesn't sleep very much at all. He just naps a lot." In fact, the assistant added, Edison's "genius for sleep equaled his genius for invention. He could go to sleep anywhere, anytime, on anything."[3]

Modern scientists and other sleep experts no longer believe that Edison, Franklin, and other purported sleep haters were true polyphasic sleepers. As one researcher, Piotr A. Wozniak, puts it, "Those polyphasic stories are very hard to confirm. Somehow, the group does not include contemporary Nobel winners, presidents, or great athletes. In other words, you cannot just e-mail a celebrity and ask. All great polyphasic sleepers are dead."[4] It appears instead that Edison and other legendary short sleepers enjoyed bragging about how little sleep they got but in reality got plenty of it by taking long naps.

Since the 1970s, scientists have conducted extensive research into sleep and how it affects human health.

What the Research Reveals

The importance of getting enough sleep, even for creative geniuses and national leaders, was proved in the last few decades or so (beginning around 1970). During that period,

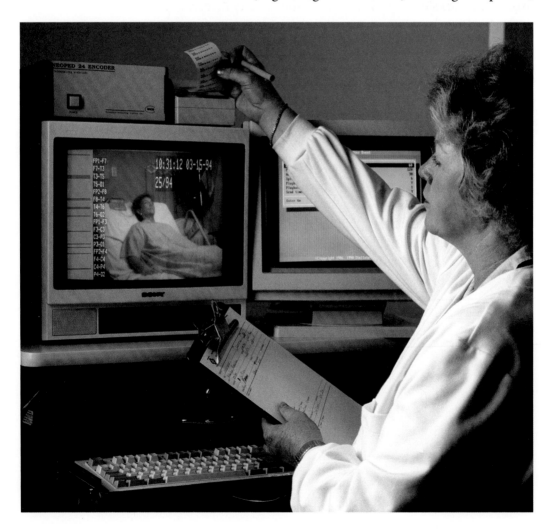

scientists conducted extensive research into sleep and how it affects human health, thereby launching the modern discipline of sleep medicine. What they learned makes it clear that, depending on the individual, getting six to eight (or occasionally more) hours of sleep a day is essential to maintaining good health, clear thinking, and creativity.

Moreover, these studies revealed that large numbers of Americans do *not* get enough sleep. Up to 58 percent experience the leading sleep disorder—insomnia—at some point in their lives. No less troubling, more than 30 million Americans—fully 10 percent of the population—suffer from one or more sleep disorders on a regular basis. A sleep disorder is a problem associated with sleep that the medical community recognizes and, when possible, diagnoses and treats.

Because so many people regularly battle such sleep problems, even those who do not do so likely know someone who does. Exposure to a relative's or friend's bad sleeping habits increases the risk that a person may develop such habits him- or herself because this person may begin keeping the same odd hours. It is therefore important for everyone to be familiar with the basic causes and symptoms of sleep disorders. As Carlos H. Schenck of the Minnesota Regional Sleep Disorders Center says, learning about these problems can also be intriguing because one gains "a glimpse into the exciting world of sleep research and the many mysteries surrounding sleep that continue to be unearthed."[5]

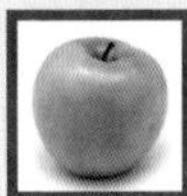

CHAPTER 1

Why Sleep Is Vital to Everyone

Whether they like it or not, all human beings—every single person on the planet—spend approximately one-third of their lives unconscious, with no clue to what is happening around them. During that period of several hours each day when they are oblivious to the world, they are asleep. Some sleep experts have remarked they find it odd that most people know so little about the causes of what is in a sense the loss of a major portion of their lives. Instead, the vast majority of people simply accept this loss as a fact of life and focus their attention on the other two-thirds of their lives—their waking hours, days, and years. One sleep expert quips:

> Considering that people on average will spend 25 years of their lives asleep, it's surprising how little most of us know about what goes on when the lights go off. It's almost as if our waking selves and sleeping selves are two separate beings living in alternate dimensions, never catching more than a passing glimpse of each other. Most people don't seem very curious or concerned about this odd desire they have to close their eyes, lie down, and blank out for several hours every night.[6]

What Is Sleep?

Fortunately for the rest of the population, a tiny band of scientists, doctors, and other researchers have devoted most or all of their lives to investigating sleep and advancing the science of sleep medicine. Their findings have revealed a great deal of information about sleep, creating a constantly growing field of data. Its contents show how sleep affects the human brain and body, how getting too little sleep can be harmful to both, what causes sleep disorders, and how these problems might be overcome. Moreover, anyone who is interested can learn these facts by reading books or online articles or watching educational television shows about sleep.

Naturally enough, the first order of business for the sleep scientists—also sometimes called sleep researchers, sleep experts, and sleep detectives—was trying to figure out exactly what sleep is. They already knew the general dictionary definitions for it. *Merriam-Webster*'s version, for example, reads: "The natural periodic suspension of consciousness during which the powers of the body are restored."[7] Because

During the course of a normal lifetime, a person spends an average of twenty-five years asleep.

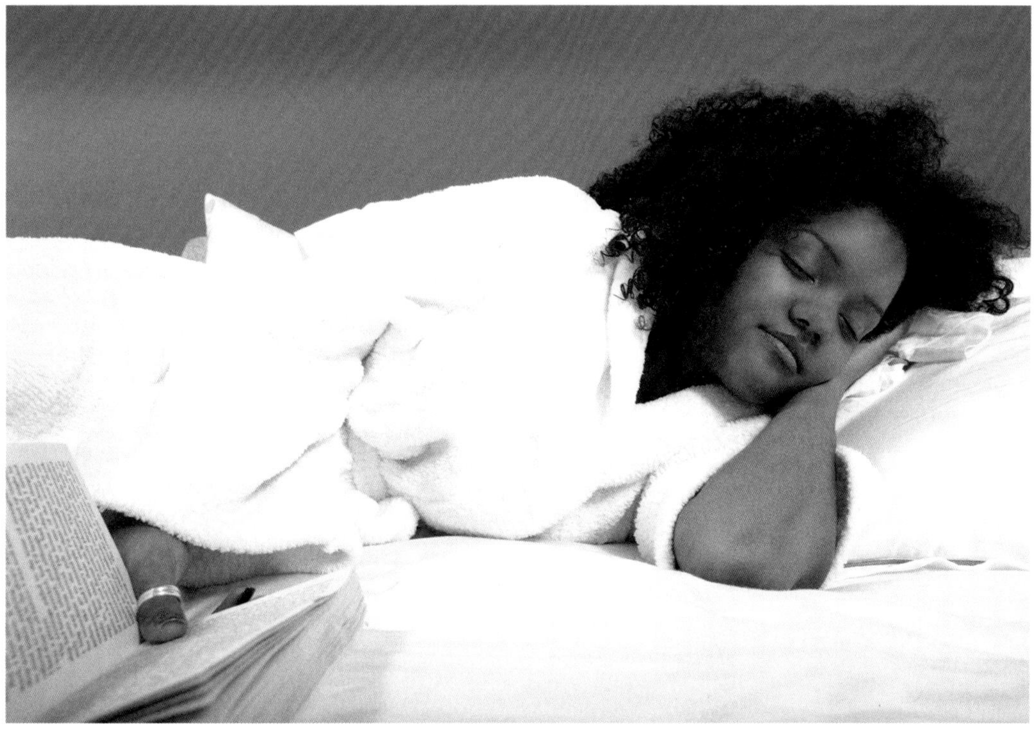

such descriptions pretty much state the obvious in simplistic terms, the researchers knew they had to be far more specific and detailed in explaining sleep.

Modern medical investigators immediately noticed one important fact about sleep. Namely, the old adage that the body and brain shut down during sleep was wrong. Indeed, in regard to the brain, just the opposite was true. During sleep the brain is quite busy as it manages numerous and diverse biological processes that get the sleeper ready for the next waking period. Health expert and editor Melinda Smith and her colleagues offer the helpful analogy of changing the oil in one's car on a regular basis: "Without enough hours of restorative sleep, you're like a car in need of an oil change. You won't be able to work, learn, create, and communicate at

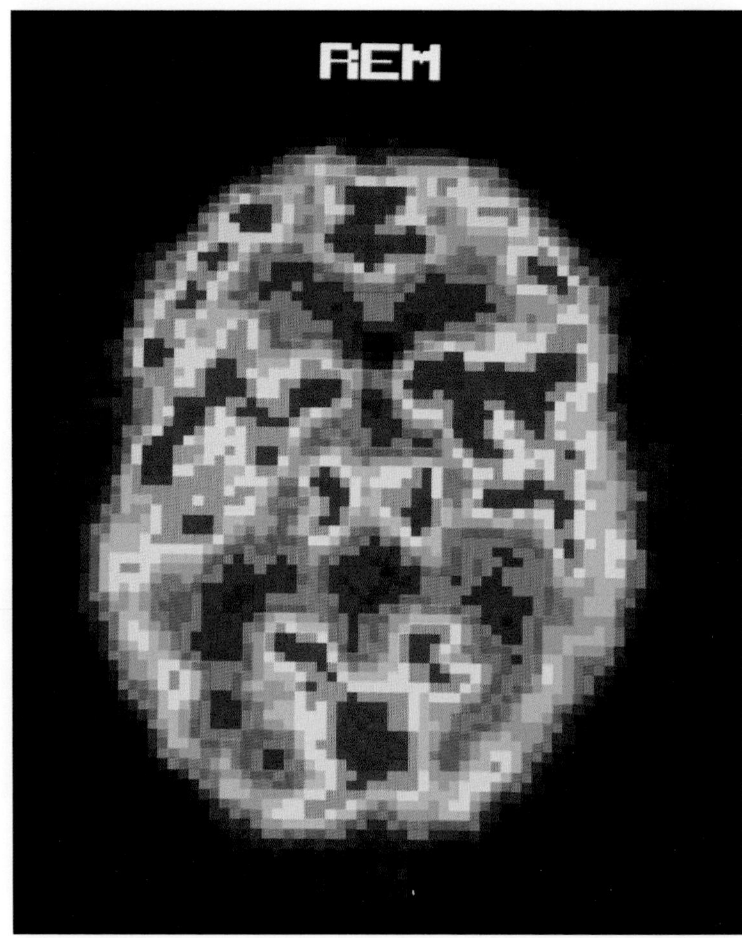

In this colored positron emission tomography (PET) scan of the human brain during sleep, active areas of the brain are shown in red whereas inactive areas are shown in blue.

a level even close to your true potential. Regularly skimp on 'service' and you're headed for a major mental and physical breakdown."[8]

Sleep detectives also learned that the number of hours required for a person's so-called daily oil change was less important than the quality of that change. In turn, the quality of sleep depends on how well the brain regulates its circadian rhythm. Also known as the biological clock, it consists of an internal twenty-four-hour cycle of wakefulness and sleep that responds to natural changes in light and darkness—that is, day and night.

HEALTH FACT

According to the National Sleep Foundation, the sleep debt a person accumulates eventually must be repaid. If someone loses an hour of sleep, he or she will need to get an extra hour later or else pay for it in some degree of reduced health.

When this sleep-wake cycle in the brain proceeds normally, one gets some high-quality sleep. In contrast, if the cycle is disrupted, the quality of sleep is diminished. Typical disruptions include waking up too often during the night, rapidly traveling through several time zones in an airplane, and regularly following a schedule of working at night and sleeping in the daytime. If such disruptions occur often, the person becomes tired, unsettled, and/or confused, and he or she can react by feeling ill at ease or being grumpy or short-tempered.

Impaired Mental Heath

Getting enough quality sleep is important, and not simply to avoid feeling tired and acting grouchy around family and friends. Sleep is absolutely vital to everyone's health because it safeguards people's mental and physical well-being, improves their quality of life, and sometimes keeps them safe from accidents and injury. In addition, getting the proper amount of good sleep supports normal growth and development in children and teens.

If a person—either a teen or an adult—fails to get enough good sleep, he or she will become sleep deficient, or sleep deprived. That can lead to various kinds of damage to one's mental and/or physical health. This impairment can happen suddenly, such as when somebody has a car crash because he or she fell asleep at the wheel. Or it can happen more gradually, such as when a person develops chronic, or persistent, mental health problems.

Such mental health problems develop because the brain requires a certain amount of good sleep to function properly, and difficulties arise when it cannot do that. For example, sleep helps the brain form new cellular links and pathways that promote learning and memory. So sleep deficiency negatively affects one's ability to remember things. It also makes it harder for a person to make decisions or solve problems.

Children who do not get enough good sleep often have trouble getting along with others and may suffer from mood swings, sudden losses of temper, or bouts of depression (prolonged, deep sadness). Quite commonly they also get lower grades in school. Finally, in extreme cases of sleep deficiency, individuals may take risks that endanger their life or may even purposely take their own life.

Percentage of high school students who received eight or more hours of sleep a night,* by sex, race/ethnicity, and grade, 2009

	Female %	Male %	Total %
Race/ethnicity			
White†	26.6	34.4	**30.8**
Black†	32.7	27.4	**30.0**
Hispanic	32.0	36.1	**34.1**
Grade			
9	36.2	42.8	**39.8**
10	28.7	33.4	**31.3**
11	25.5	27.7	**26.6**
12	21.3	27.1	**24.2**
Total %	**28.2**	**33.3**	**30.9**

*On an average school night
†Non-Hispanic

SOURCE: Centers for Disease Control and Prevention. Youth Risk Behavior Surveillance—United States, 2009. Surveillance Summaries, June 4, 2010. *MMWR* 2010; 59 (No. SS-5).

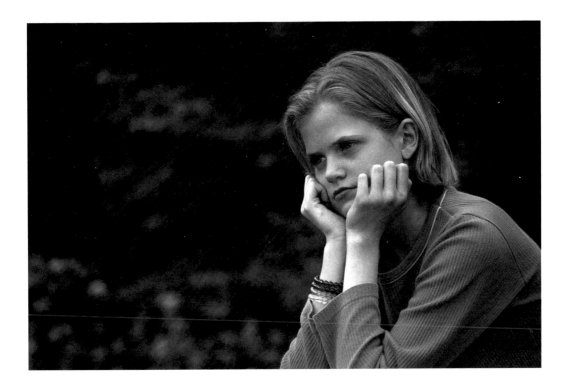

Impacts on Physical Health

Children who do not get enough sleep often have trouble getting along with others and may suffer mood swings, temper tantrums, and bouts of depression.

On the flip side—in regard to sleep's role in maintaining good *physical* health—getting a decent amount of good sleep keeps all sorts of bodily systems and processes running smoothly. One of these processes is the one in which the heart and blood vessels regularly repair themselves. According to researchers at Harvard Medical School's Division of Sleep Medicine, one of sleep's more important tasks

> is to give the heart a chance to rest from the constant demands of waking life. As compared to wakefulness, during [some stages of] sleep there is an overall reduction in heart rate and blood pressure. During [deep] sleep, however, there is a more pronounced variation in cardiovascular [circulatory] activity, with overall increases in blood pressure and heart rate. . . . The underlying reason for these considerable neural and physiological variations in [deep] sleep is currently unknown, and may be a by-product of . . . changes in nervous system activity or related to dream content.[9]

By contrast, doctors have linked getting too *little* sleep to increased risks of high blood pressure, heart disease, stroke, and diabetes. In addition, the risk of obesity seems to be higher in people who suffer from sleep deficiency. According to the National Heart, Lung, and Blood Institute (NHLBI):

> One study of teenagers showed that with each hour of sleep lost, the odds of becoming obese went up. Sleep deficiency increases the risk of obesity in other age groups as well. Sleep helps maintain a healthy balance of the hormones that make you feel hungry (ghrelin) or full (leptin). When you don't get enough sleep, your level of ghrelin goes up and your level of leptin goes down. This makes you feel hungrier than when you're well-rested.[10]

Another aspect of physical health supported by getting enough good sleep is normal bodily growth. When a person experiences deep sleep, the body releases a hormone that encourages cell, organ, and bone growth in children and teens. This hormone also expands muscle mass and aids in cell and tissue repair.

The human immune system is also directly impacted by the amount of good sleep a person gets. The immune system mounts a vigorous defense against germs and other harmful substances that enter the body. So a person who is experiencing sleep deficiency may not be able to effectively fend off even some of the minor infections, like the common cold, that threaten one's health from time to time.

Because these and other bodily systems and processes depend to one degree or another on sleep, a prolonged lack of good sleep can cause an overall reduction in the body's health. In turn, that can make a person both feel and be less productive, as well as take longer to complete normal tasks. Sleep deficiency can also cause someone to display slower reaction times to outside stimuli and make more mistakes, including while operating dangerous machinery or driving a car or truck. The Centers for Disease Control and Prevention (CDC) sums up the physical risks of getting too little sleep:

> Insufficient sleep is associated with a number of chronic diseases and conditions—such as diabetes, cardio-

vascular disease, obesity, and depression—which threaten our nation's health. Notably, insufficient sleep is associated with the onset of these diseases and also poses important implications for their management and outcome. Moreover, insufficient sleep is responsible for motor vehicle and machinery-related crashes, causing substantial injury and disability each year. In short, drowsy driving can be as dangerous—and preventable—as driving while intoxicated.[11]

Normal Sleep Stages

The kind of sleep required to avoid sleep deficiency has been variously described as "high quality," "good," "deep," and "decent." These are general, nonclinical terms, however. Scientists, doctors, and other sleep researchers use more-technical terms to describe sleep. Moreover, they point out that several different kinds, or stages, of sleep exist and that these stages are considerably different from one another in the manner in which they affect the brain and ultimately the body as a whole.

First, the experts say, there are two main types of sleep—REM and non-REM. The letters of the acronym *REM* stand for "rapid eye movement," a reference to the fact that a person's eyes move back and forth quickly during this stage. Four non-REM sleep stages exist, each one deeper than the one before it. The fifth stage, REM sleep, is the one in which most dreaming occurs.

A sleeping individual typically spends about 75 percent of his or her night in non-REM sleep. The first stage consists of the blurry, shadowy, hard-to-define period that lies between being awake and aware of what is happening and being asleep and mostly *un*aware. Stage one of non-REM sleep is therefore best described as light sleep.

In non-REM sleep's second stage, sometimes called the "baseline" of sleep, the sleeper becomes still less aware of his or her surroundings. The person's heart rate slows somewhat, and his or her temperature drops slightly, although

HEALTH FACT

The NHLBI says that sleepy drivers cause roughly one hundred thousand car accidents each year, resulting in approximately fifteen hundred deaths.

breathing remains regular. The third stage of sleep follows. Experts often call it "delta sleep" because the brain begins to produce invisible electromagnetic emissions known as delta waves.

Next comes stage four of non-REM sleep, the one directly preceding REM sleep itself. Like stage three, stage four witnesses the production of delta waves, but it is during this fourth stage that the body's most numerous restorative activities occur. Blood supplies to the muscles increase and the body's tissues readily grow and repair themselves. Also, hormones, including the one essential for muscle and bone growth, are released. "It's a common misconception," Schenck explains,

> that REM sleep is the deepest sleep. Actually, stage 4 non-REM is the deepest sleep, closely followed by stage 3. When you've been sleep deprived, your body craves delta sleep and will try to make up for lost time by getting you to stage 4 faster and keeping you there longer. When people say that someone is "out like a light" or in a "dead sleep," the person is probably in stage 3 or 4, when it's very difficult to arouse someone. This is the stage from which sleep terrors and sleepwalking are most likely to occur. Stage 4 is also the stage, it's thought, when the body does most of its repair work.[12]

Finally comes REM sleep, in which the sleeper spends about 25 percent of his or her nightly sleep session. REM sleep usually first sets in roughly ninety minutes after falling asleep, and it is not necessarily the only stage that occurs thereafter. In fact, it is not unusual for a sleeper to slip back and forth from REM sleep to stage four, then to stage two, then back to stage three, four, and REM, then to stage four again, and so forth throughout the rest of the sleep session. During REM sleep, which is almost as deep as stages three and four, the brain and body gain energy and are refreshed. Most strikingly, while the eyes dart back and forth, dreams occur. In addition, REM sleep is essential to both learning and memory. During REM sleep, the brain somehow processes the information the person took in, via seeing and

Some Mammals Sleep Differently

Sleep researchers have determined that most animals—and all mammals—sleep on a regular, usually daily basis. Not all mammals sleep in the same manner, however, as explained here by the medical team at Harvard Medical School's Division of Sleep Medicine.

> In all mammals and many other animals, sleep can be defined in much the same way that we define sleep for humans. However, there are some notable differences among species. When humans sleep, the entire brain is involved. Dolphins and whales, on the other hand, need to maintain consciousness while they sleep so they can occasionally surface to breathe. In these marine mammals, sleep occurs in only one hemisphere of their brain at a time—allowing for some degree of consciousness and vigilance to be maintained at all times.

Stuart F. Quan, ed. "The Characteristics of Sleep." Healthy Sleep, December 18, 2007. http://healthysleep.med.harvard.edu/healthy/science/what/characteristics.

Most mammals sleep on a regular basis.

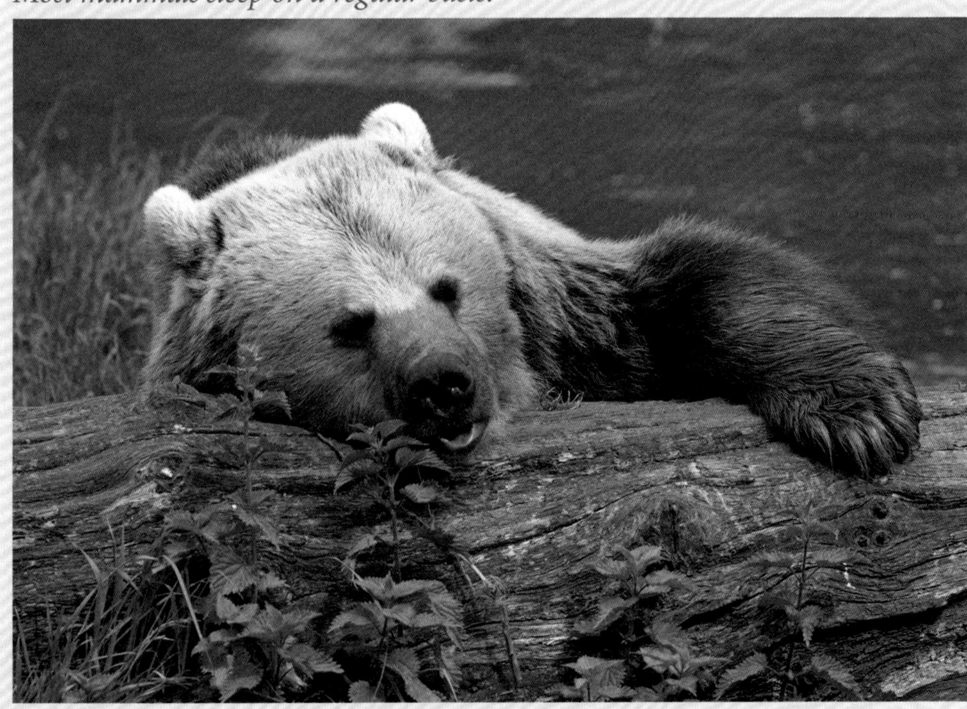

hearing, during the previous day. This processing helps create new brain-cell connections that strengthen and sharpen a person's memory.

How Much Sleep?

Evidence shows that the amount of sleep required for restfulness and good health does vary somewhat from person to person. Still, the range of hours involved is not very large. According to the National Institutes of Health (NIH), most healthy adults need approximately seven to nine hours of sleep a night to function at their peak performance. Children and teens need more—approximately eight to ten hours per night—and babies still more, up to fifteen hours or more. A common myth claims that seniors (people in their mid-fifties and older) need less and less sleep as they age. The reality, however, is that older people still require between seven and eight hours of sleep per night. (One common way elderly folk get the sleep they need is to sleep four or five hours at night and make up the shortfall by taking one or two naps in the daytime.)

Recommended hours of sleep, by age group

Infants	
0–2 months	12–18 hours
2–12 months	14–15 hours
Toddlers/Children	
1–3 years	12–14 hours
3–5 years	11–13 hours
5–10 years	10–11 hours
Adolescents	
10–17 years	8.5–9.25 hours
Adults	
18+	7–9 hours

SOURCE: National Sleep Foundation. "How Much Sleep Do We Really Need?" www.sleepfoundation.org/article/how-sleep-works/how-much-sleep-do-we-really-need.

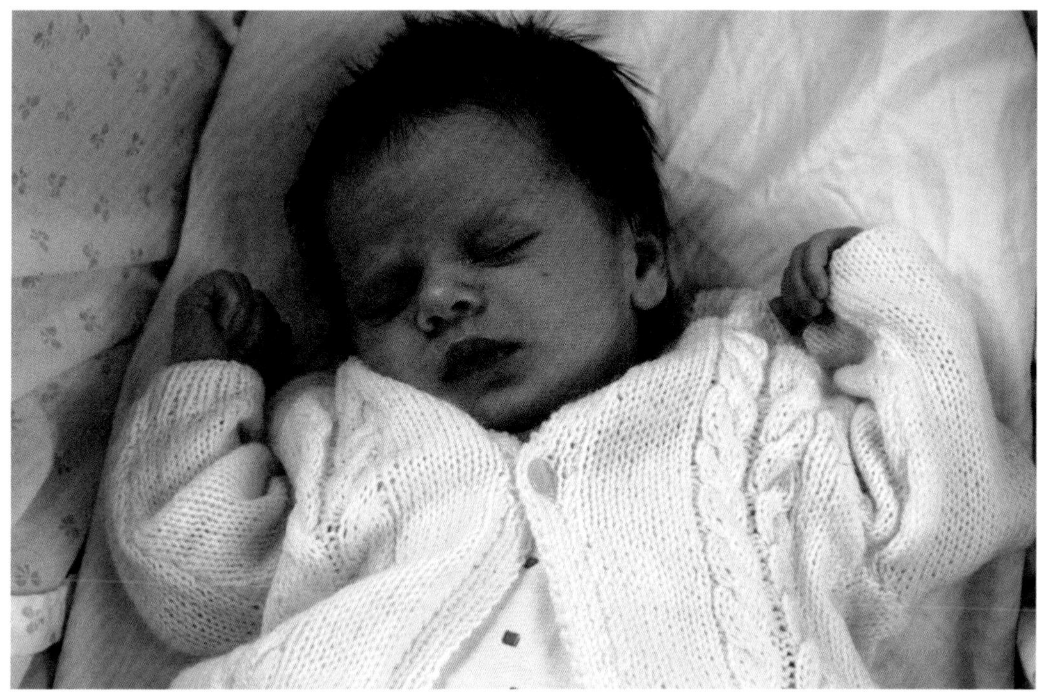

Some people think that these recommendations are wrong. They may be convinced that they can somehow avoid getting their recommended amount of sleep and still maintain excellent health. A number of them claim that they get by fine on just six hours of sleep per night, and apparently at least a few of them are correct. Researchers at the University of California–San Francisco recently discovered a gene that allows a person to function normally on only six hours of sleep a night. *USA Today*'s Elizabeth Weise reports:

Most healthy adults need seven to nine hours of sleep to function optimally, whereas children and teens need eight to ten hours, and babies need fifteen hours or more.

> The mutation [altered gene] seems to result in people who are natural short sleepers, needing much less than the normal eight [or more hours] that most humans require for well-rested functioning. . . . [The researchers] were able to genetically engineer both fruit flies and mice to have the same mutation and have been researching its causes and effects. It appears that humans and mice that carry the mutation get more intense sleep, as measured by slow-wave electrical activity in the brain, and so need less of it.[13]

The problem, the researchers found, is that very few people have the gene in question. Indeed, less than 3 percent of the people in the United States carry it. That means that the other 97 percent of the population require more than six hours of sleep a night to remain in optimum health. "So," Weise adds, "almost everyone who claims they only need six hours of sleep are kidding themselves."[14]

It also means that, for the average person, routine sleep loss adds up and has negative consequences. The total sleep a person loses in a night, two nights, a week, or more is called "sleep debt." In some ways it resembles one's monetary debt. If someone withdraws two dollars a day from his or her bank account, at the end of one week the account will be short fourteen dollars. If the person needs all the money that was originally in the account to pay bills, he or she will have to deposit fourteen dollars back into the account. Similarly, if a person loses two hours of sleep a night for a week, he or she will have a sleep debt of fourteen hours. To stay alert and healthy, the person will need to replace those hours sooner or later.

Symptoms of Sleep Deprivation

Unfortunately for a lot of Americans, they owe quite a lot of debt to the sleep bank, so to speak, and on a regular basis. The NIH, CDC, and other leading health organizations say that the average American adult sleeps less than seven hours a night. "In today's fast-paced society, six or seven hours of sleep may sound pretty good," Smith and her colleagues write. But "in reality it's a recipe for chronic sleep deprivation."[15] Indeed, according to sleep experts, people who regularly get less than eight hours of sleep a night are sleep deprived whether they realize it or not. Furthermore, they frequently have no clue as to how much that sleep debt negatively affects their life.

One reason that someone may not be aware of how a lack of sleep has changed his or her life is that the symptoms of sleep deprivation are often less obvious than one might expect. Another reason is that the person may be so used to sleep deprivation that he or she may not recall how it feels to be well rested and fully alert. The "new normal" of his or her life gives the impression that feeling groggy at certain times of the day is to be expected by everyone. The reality, however, is that such feelings are normal only for those who are chronically sleep deprived.

Leading health organizations and sleep clinics say that certain habits and feelings that occur daily or quite frequently in someone's life may be signs of mild sleep deprivation. One such habit is having a difficult time getting out of bed in the morning, *every* morning. Needing to set an alarm clock and requiring the use of a snooze button to wake up on time every morning may be another sign.

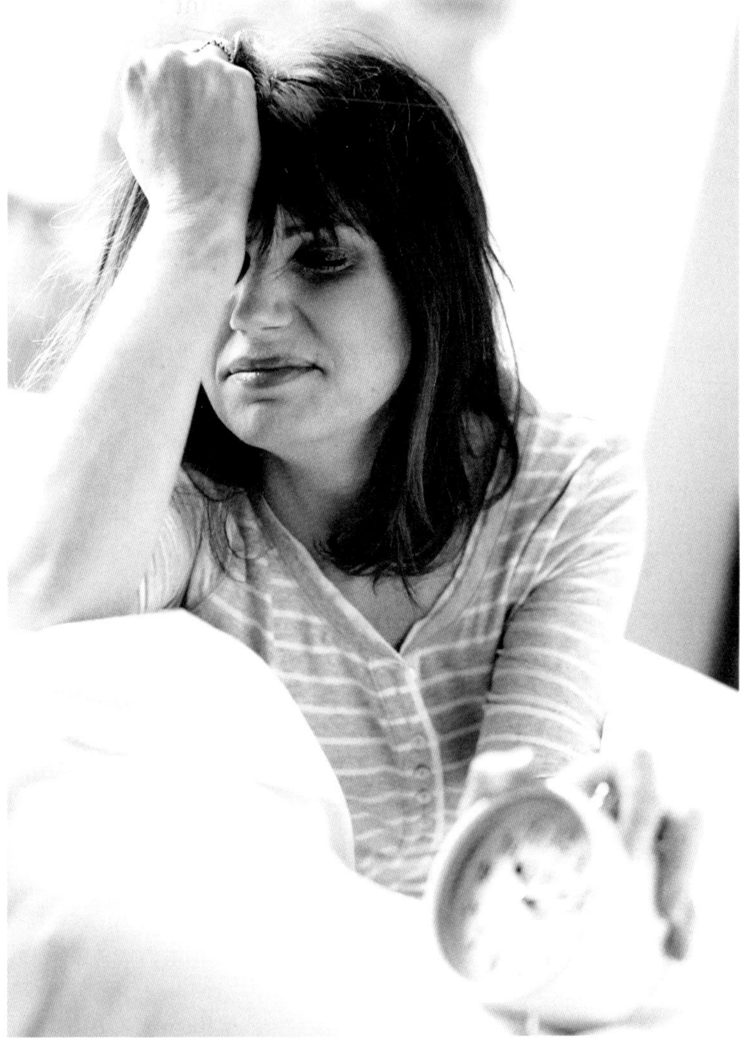

One sign of sleep deprivation is difficulty getting out of bed every morning.

Outsmarting That Pesky Alarm

Few adults with jobs and other responsibilities feel they can function normally without an alarm clock to wake them up each morning. But that device can be a pesky nuisance that interrupts one's healthy sleep cycles. Health expert and editor Melinda Smith and her colleagues give the following advice on how to outsmart the alarm clock:

> Even if you've enjoyed a full night's sleep, getting out of bed can be difficult if your alarm goes off when you're in the middle of deep sleep (stage N3). If you want to make mornings less painful—or if you know you only have a limited time for sleep—try setting a wake-up time that's a multiple of 90 minutes, the length of the average sleep cycle. For example, if you go to bed at 10 p.m., set your alarm for 5:30 (a total of 7½ hours of sleep) instead of 6:00 or 6:30. You may feel more refreshed at 5:30 than with another 30 to 60 minutes of sleep because you're getting up at the end of a sleep cycle when your body and brain are already close to wakefulness.

Melinda Smith, Lawrence Robinson, and Robert Segal. "How Much Sleep Do You Need?" Helpguide. www.helpguide.org/life/sleeping.htm.

Experiencing small bouts of tiredness in the midafternoon, while driving, in meetings at work or in school, after a heavy meal, or in warm rooms could be another indication that someone is sleep deprived. Still another warning sign is dozing off while watching television, attending a movie, or reading a book.

The longer someone goes without sleep, the bigger his or her sleep debt becomes. Symptoms of more serious sleep deprivation include feeling glum, irritable, or moody; experiencing weariness or exhaustion, as well as a lack of motivation for doing standard activities; having less ability to solve problems or express creativity than in the past; catching colds more easily and more often than in the past; having a reduced ability to deal with stress; experiencing unusual weight gain that makes the person uncomfortable; having trouble concentrating and/or remembering things; having less hand-eye coordination than in the past; having increased trouble making decisions; and experiencing the onset of frequent health problems, including manifestations of diabetes, heart disease, and stroke.

Knowledge Is the Key

A sleep-deprived individual may also suffer from one or more sleep disorders and related problems. In addition to the most common one, insomnia, a few of the others include sleep apnea (stopping breathing while asleep), hypopnea (unusually shallow breathing while asleep), sleepwalking, nocturia (having to go to the bathroom repeatedly during the night), narcolepsy (suddenly falling asleep when not in bed), and night terrors (sudden, unexplained fears during one's nightly sleep session).

As is true in so many other aspects of life, the first and foremost key to dealing with and overcoming these and other sleep disorders is knowledge. A person has to know about them before he or she can confront them. As William Dement of Stanford University's sleep disorders center says:

> Almost all sleep disorders can be effectively treated or cured, and there is absolutely no reason to suffer needlessly. Unfortunately, the vast majority of sleep disorders victims *do* suffer needlessly because most people do not know about sleep disorders. . . . Millions of people are suffering and thousands are dying each year without ever knowing the true cause of their problems. [That is why learning] about sleep and dreams, the nature and consequences of sleep deprivation, and common sleep disorder symptoms is essential.[16]

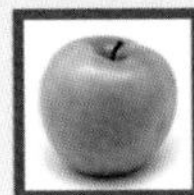
CHAPTER **2**

The Chief Sleep Disorder: Insomnia

"Your husband snores" and "your kids are up half the night," a medical editor for *U.S. News & World Report* writes, directly addressing the typical American woman suffering from insomnia.

> You're worried about a big presentation at work. It's no surprise you have insomnia. The real shocker would be not feeling tired at the start of the day. A 2007 National Sleep Foundation (NSF) survey found that nearly two thirds of women said they got a good night's sleep only a few nights a week; 29 percent took sleeping pills or other sleep aids regularly. Eighty percent said they don't slow down when they're tired. Most just prop their eyes open and get through the day.[17]

A Major Medical Problem

As the National Sleep Foundation's 2007 study showed, insomnia is a major medical problem affecting an exceptionally large proportion of Americans. The exact number of people in the country who "get through the day" in a semi-groggy state is unknown. But the National Sleep Foundation and other leading authorities on sleep problems estimate that up to 22 percent of the population, or some 70 million Americans, experience insomnia almost every night. No less staggering, about 48 percent, or some 150 million Americans, suffer from insomnia's symptoms on occasion. That the above statement from *U.S. News & World Report* is addressed specifically to women reflects the fact that they experience it more often than men do. For reasons that are still unclear, for every ten male insomniacs, there are an estimated thirteen female ones.

Whether a man or a woman, in simple terms, someone who has insomnia has difficulty falling asleep, staying asleep, or both. In addition, even after she or he manages to nod off, often it is not a very good or refreshing sleep. So on awakening, the person may still feel tired. Moreover, insomnia can bring on feelings of drowsiness and listlessness during the daytime. It is not unusual for an insomniac to feel irritable or depressed and to have difficulty paying attention and remembering things. In turn, this can negatively affect

Up to 22 percent of the U.S. population suffers from disordered sleep, which constitutes a major medical problem.

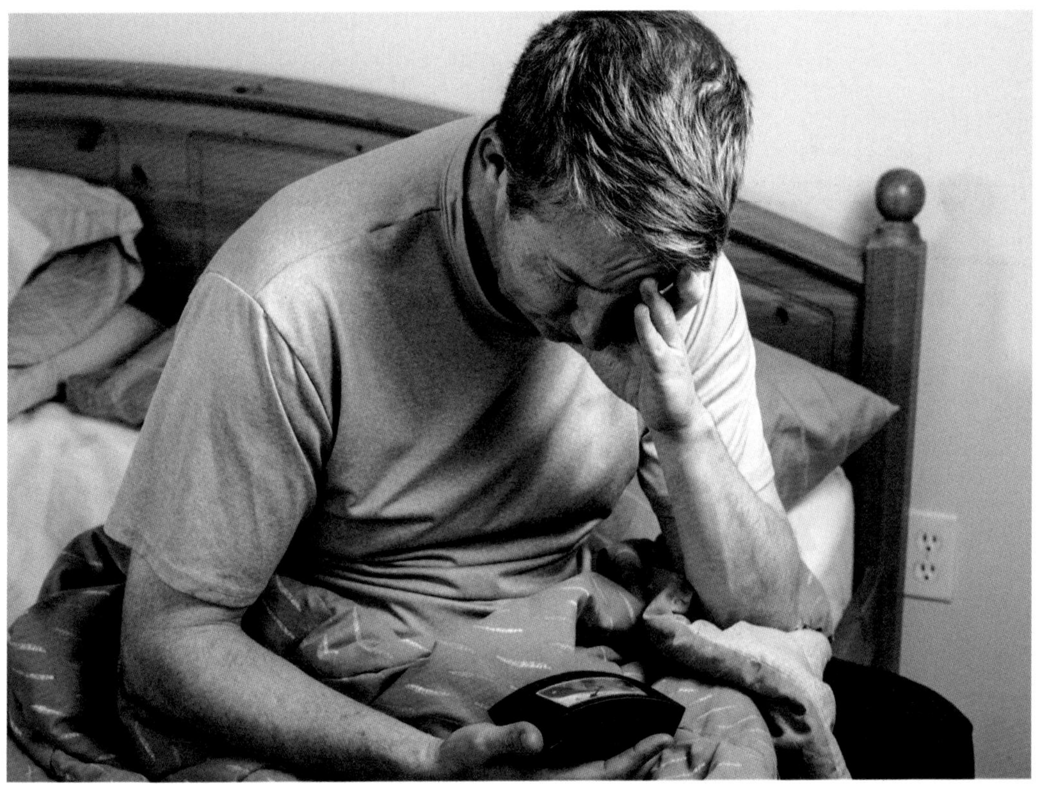

one's performance at work or in school. The disorder can be dangerous, too, such as when an insomniac becomes sleepy while driving and as a result has a serious accident.

Finally, insomnia costs the country an immense amount of money each year, funds that could otherwise go to pay for more positive, constructive endeavors. In 2011, according to a Harvard Medical School study, the direct cost of insomnia to the U.S. economy was $63.2 billion. "This figure," noted Baylor University scholar Max Hirshkowitz says,

> includes the cost for both prescription and over the counter (OTC) sleep medications, visits to healthcare providers, and nursing home care to treat insomnia in elderly patients. In addition, insomnia also produces a number of indirect costs. These costs result from lower economic output due to symptoms produced by insomnia that affect job performance, such as increased absenteeism, impaired memory and concentration, decreased ability to complete daily tasks, and decreased problem-solving abilities.[18]

Different Kinds of Insomnia

Because of these and other damaging costs to society, in the past few decades medical experts have poured a lot of time and effort into studying insomnia. They learned who is most at risk for the condition. They also determined its many symptoms and learned a great deal about what causes it. These studies revealed that women are not the only members of society who are particularly at risk for insomnia. Elderly people, for instance, are more likely to experience the condition than younger individuals. The NHLBI lists some other high-risk societal and economic groups, including

> those who have a lot of stress; are depressed or have other emotional distress, such as divorce or death of a spouse; have lower incomes; work at night or have frequent major shifts in their work hours; travel long distances with time changes; have certain medical conditions or sleep disorders that can disrupt sleep

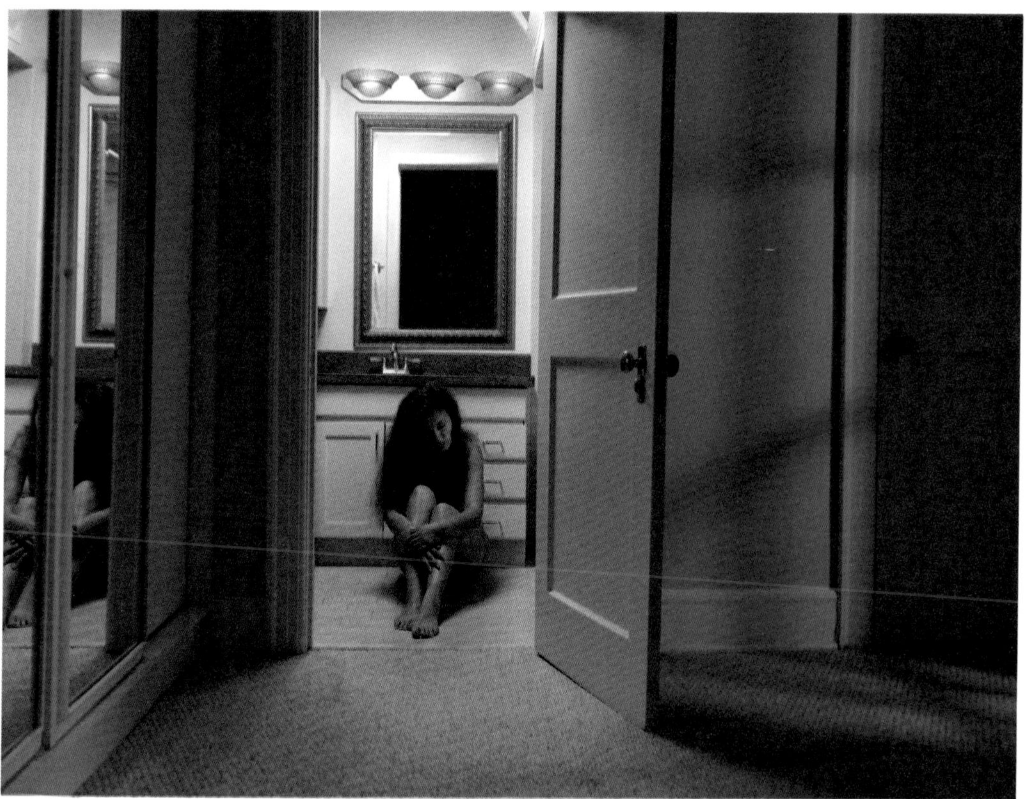

People with insomnia have a difficult time falling asleep, staying asleep, or both.

> [and/or] have an inactive lifestyle. Young and middle-aged African Americans also might be at increased risk for insomnia. Research shows that, compared with Caucasian Americans, it takes African Americans longer to fall asleep. They also have lighter sleep [and] don't sleep as well.[19]

Whether they are in these high-risk groups or not, those who get insomnia suffer from distinct kinds. Medical authorities define these categories according to different criteria, one being how long the condition lasts. Insomnia can be short-term (also called acute or transient insomnia), for example. People with short-term insomnia usually experience sleeplessness from a single night up to a few weeks, and then they return to normal sleep patterns. In contrast, a person who experiences insomnia three or more nights a week for a month or longer is said to have chronic, or long-term, insomnia.

HEALTH FACT

The CDC says that more than one-quarter of the U.S. population report sometimes not getting enough sleep and that almost 10 percent report experiencing regular bouts of insomnia.

Medical experts also define the condition as either primary or secondary insomnia, depending on what causes it. Primary insomnia is a medical condition and sleep disorder in and of itself, with various causes that remain only partially understood. As Hirshkowitz says, "All sleeplessness that isn't due to a medical, psychiatric, neurological, or environmental cause is called primary insomnia, meaning the insomnia itself *is* the medical condition and isn't just a symptom of something else."[20] Secondary insomnia is different in that it is a symptom of some other medical problem or caused by common household sounds such as a baby crying or a faucet leaking.

Typical Symptoms

Whatever kind of insomnia a person may have, the symptoms are usually the same or similar. First and foremost, he or she has trouble falling asleep. The person may also wake up fairly frequently during the night and have difficulty getting back to sleep, as well as wake up earlier than necessary or desired the next morning. Furthermore, the insomniac feels tired or drowsy almost every morning, no matter when he or she wakes up.

Nancy Foldvary-Schaefer, director of the Sleep Disorders Center at the Cleveland Clinic, lists some other common symptoms of insomnia, framing them in the form of questions, as she would to her patients.

> Do you notice that although you have difficulty falling asleep at night, you fall asleep easily during sedentary [seated] activities, such as watching television or reading? Do you watch television, read, or eat in bed? Are you a worrywart? Does your mind race at night? Do you spend the nighttime hours thinking about your problems, the next day's schedule, or worries about sleep loss? Do you experience increased muscle ten-

sion or agitation . . . or inability to relax at night? Have you experienced a recent life change or emotional stress? Do you feel anxious [or] grow tired or irritable, or feel a deterioration of mood or motivation, during the day?[21]

Another common symptom of insomnia, which can be highly problematic, is feeling drowsy while driving a car, truck, or other motor vehicle. Tiredness while behind the wheel causes many thousands of serious car accidents each year, a number of which prove fatal for the driver and/or others involved in the crash. Similarly, studies indicate that insomnia significantly increases the risk of elderly folk, especially women, falling down and injuring themselves. According to Phyllis C. Zee, director of the

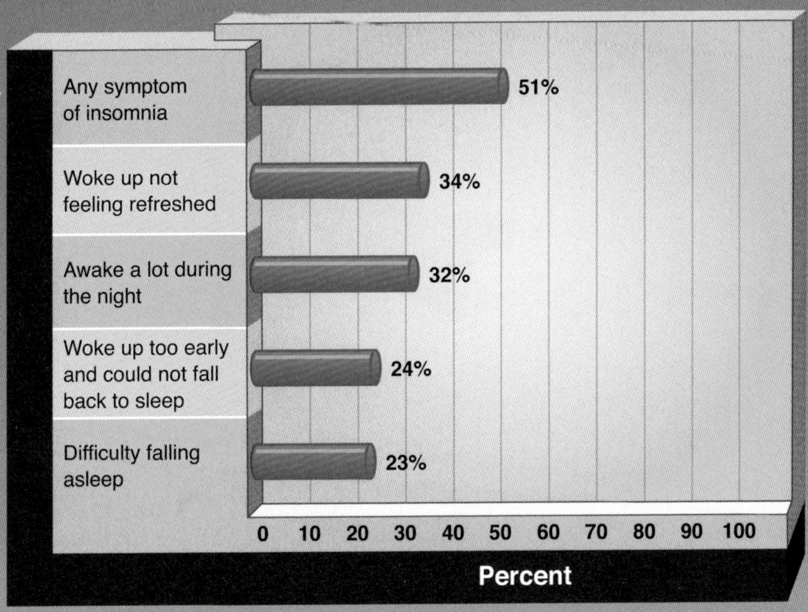

Taken from: National Sleep Foundation. www.sleepfoundation.org.

The Same as Being Drunk

Having chronic insomnia can be dangerous. According to a study published by the British journal *Occupational and Environmental Medicine* in 2000, researchers in Australia and New Zealand found that regularly getting too little sleep can produce many of the same harmful effects as being drunk. A health report released that same year by CNN summarized the findings, saying:

> Getting less than 6 hours a night can affect coordination, reaction time and judgment, posing "a very serious risk." Drivers are especially vulnerable, the researchers warned. They found that people who drive after being awake for 17 to 19 hours performed worse than those with a blood alcohol level of .05 percent. That's the legal limit for drunk driving in most western European countries . . . . The study said 16 to 60 percent of road accidents involve sleep deprivation. The researchers said countries with drunk driving laws should consider similar restrictions against sleep-deprived driving.

CNN.com. "Sleep Deprivation as Bad as Alcohol Impairment, Study Suggests," September 20, 2000. http://archives.cnn.com/2000/HEALTH/09/20/sleep.deprivation.

Sleep-deprived persons often drive less skillfully than drivers who have been drinking.

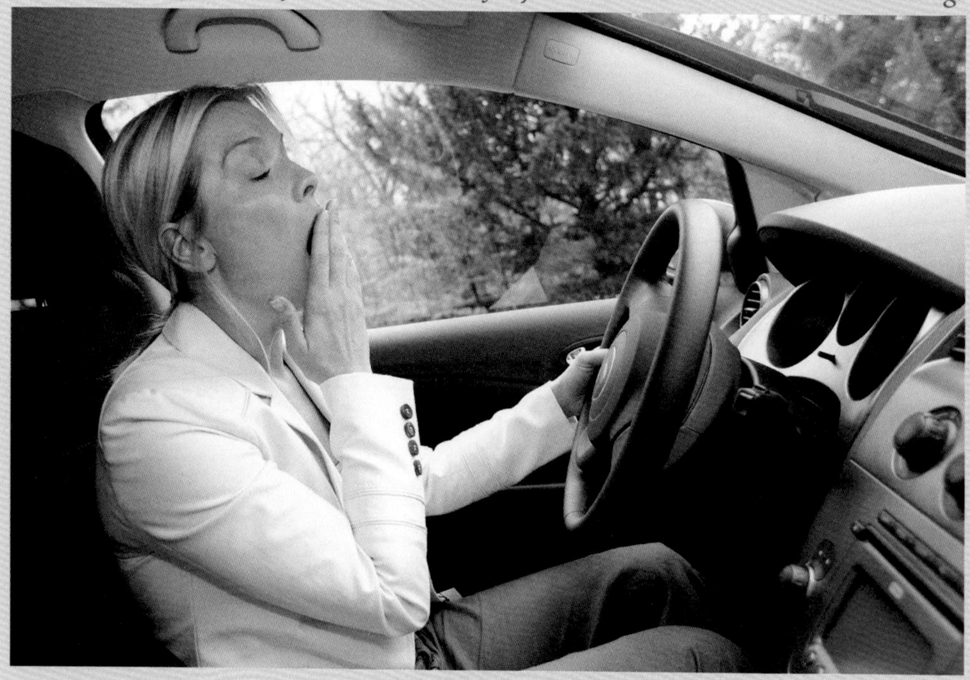

Sleep Disorders Center at Northwestern Memorial Hospital in Chicago:

> Nighttime sleep problems are a significant risk factor for falls in the elderly. More recently, results from a large study suggested that the underlying insomnia, rather than the medications used to treat it, increased the risk for falls in elderly nursing home residents. The investigators found that untreated or partially treated residents with insomnia had a higher risk for falls than those who take sleep medications to improve their sleep. In older people, there are multiple mental and physical factors that, when combined with insomnia, can lead to falls.[22]

Stress and Other Triggers

No less important than recognizing the symptoms of insomnia is determining the causes of the condition. Research conducted by doctors, hospitals, and sleep centers has confirmed a number of reasons why people suffer from this irritating and at times debilitating problem. Primary insomnia—the kind that is not a symptom of another disorder—can be triggered by stress, for example. (Medical authorities think that stress is a physical or mental reaction to positive or negative situations in a person's life.) Minor stress, like the kind a person quite naturally feels when one is late for work, might cause acute, or short-term, insomnia. When the stress is more serious and prolonged over the course of months or even years, however, the result can be chronic insomnia. Serious stress can itself have numerous triggers, including repeated money troubles, the death of a loved one, divorce, job loss, and others.

Whether the stress is short-term or prolonged, typically the person is too upset to sleep, or at least to sleep as long and restfully as usual. Herbert Ross, founder of Colorado's Aspen Sleep Institute, explains why. "Stress and pent-up emotional issues," he says,

> can wreak havoc on the brain, deregulating brain chemicals and organs that are instrumental in procuring a good night's rest. Unmanaged daily stress can deplete

your hormonal and nutrient reserves and create a vicious cycle of less sleep and more stress. Additionally, unresolved psychological issues, such as deep-seated internal fears or relationship conflicts, can disturb brain chemistry and hinder deep sleep.[23]

Other causes of primary insomnia may include medications, including some used to treat hay fever or some food allergies. Jet lag when traveling long distances in airplanes also seems to interfere with sleep. An illness can also cause insomnia by throwing off a person's sleep schedule. In addition, many experts believe that environmental factors such as too much noise or extremes of temperature can bring on bouts of insomnia. However, there is some disagreement in the medical community on this point. Stanford's William Dement argues:

> People soon habituate [get used] to repeated, meaningless noise and tend not to wake up. When my wife and I first moved to New York . . . our apartment was right next to the elevated railway. The screeching brakes of the trains entering the station kept me up much of the first night. In the morning I was incensed. "Why didn't the landlord tell me about this," I fumed. "Now we'll have to move!" But by the next night I was both seriously sleep deprived and somewhat habituated to the sound of the brakes. I slept much better that night and just fine most nights thereafter, although the trains kept on screeching.[24]

Dement is therefore skeptical of the idea that environmental factors are often direct causes of insomnia. Nevertheless, he suggests that they *can* negatively affect someone's sleep under certain special conditions. For example, he says, "if you feel that the noise is being made maliciously and deliberately to annoy you, it is likely that your sleep will be very disturbed."[25]

Depression, Pain, and Addictive Substances

Unlike primary insomnia, secondary insomnia is not itself a condition or disorder, but rather a symptom or side effect

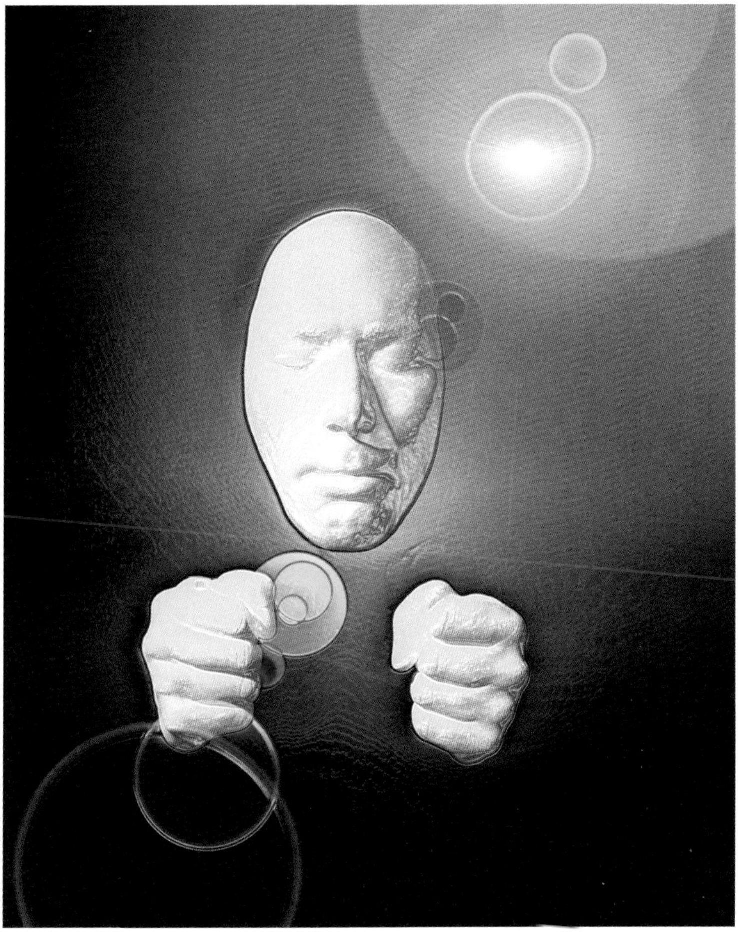

Research has confirmed that stress can cause insomnia.

of another problem. So a person who experiences secondary insomnia already suffers from an existing condition of some kind. Examples of such existing problems are emotional and sleep-related disorders, diseases and other medical conditions (including related pain), and use of certain potentially addictive substances.

Of the emotional problems that have insomnia as a byproduct, clinical depression is one of the most common and debilitating. Someone who is clinically depressed often has feelings of helplessness and hopelessness, as well as unusually low energy levels. He or she may also lose interest in daily activities or even in life itself. Among the many documented causes of depression are extreme loneliness, childhood trauma or abuse, and persistent alcohol and drug abuse. A person who has undergone such hardships and has become depressed as a result frequently has trouble sleeping. As is true of other conditions of which insomnia is a symptom, when someone who is depressed cannot sleep well, he or she must first deal with the depression itself before addressing the insomnia.

Among the medical conditions that can cause a person to suffer from insomnia are Alzheimer's disease, Parkinson's disease, and conditions that produce chronic pain,

Insomnia as a Self-Fulfilling Prophecy

As explained here by Nancy Foldvary-Schaefer, director of the Sleep Disorders Center at the Cleveland Clinic, in some cases the fear of insomnia becomes a self-fulfilling prophecy and actually triggers a kind of insomnia called psychophysiological insomnia.

> Ann is a classic case of psychophysiological insomnia. Some of the typical features of this form of insomnia are: Excessive focus on sleep or heightened anxiety levels about sleep, difficulty falling asleep in bed at the desired time [and] mental arousal in bed (racing thoughts, inability to turn off an active mind). Ann reacted to stress by not sleeping. Her pattern evolved into a lifestyle of losing sleep, and the fatigue further affected her mood and outlook. Soon, bedtime was a greater stress than the emotional tension in her life, and sleeping became an impossible feat—something she feared each night. Individuals with psychophysiological insomnia . . . blame insomnia for their lack of sleep, rather than correctly placing responsibility [on] the events currently taking place in their lives. Insomnia becomes learned, and a vicious cycle develops.

Nancy Foldvary-Schaefer. *The Cleveland Clinic Guide to Sleep Disorders*. New York: Kaplan, 2009, pp. 118–119.

like arthritis. Suffering from almost constant pain can easily interfere with normal sleeping habits. Not surprisingly, conditions that make it hard to breathe—asthma, for instance—can also impede restful sleep. In addition, heartburn and other gastrointestinal problems generate pain and discomfort that make it hard to sleep.

Still another example is menopause. Consisting of the combined bodily changes a woman undergoes in midlife when she can no longer produce the eggs necessary for having children, it is often accompanied by hot flashes, night sweats, and other severe discomforts. A woman undergoing menopause may have more than just trouble getting to sleep. She may also wake up several times during the night.

Potentially addictive substances that are known to cause insomnia include stimulants, such as caffeine and nicotine, and alcohol and other sedatives. Foldvary-Schaefer warns:

> Caffeinated substances, including coffee, tea, soda, and chocolate . . . stimulate the nervous system and may cause difficulty falling asleep or cause you to wake up during the night. This is not to say you should take your morning coffee off the breakfast menu or forget your late-afternoon chocolate. Consuming moderate amounts of caffeine during the day will not affect sleep onset in the evening for most people . . . [but] if you suffer from insomnia, limit your intake of caffeinated beverages after noon. Excessive caffeine use can lead to withdrawal symptoms, which can also affect a person's ability to sleep.[26]

Similarly, the highly addictive substance nicotine, which is found in tobacco products, can interfere with sleep. Nicotine "is a stimulant," one expert observer points out.

> It arouses and excites the nervous system. This explains why insomnia ranks high among the complaints voiced by smokers. Nicotine can affect sleep in two ways. First, since nicotine is a central nervous system stimulant, it produces almost the same effects on the body as caffeine. . . . The second way in which

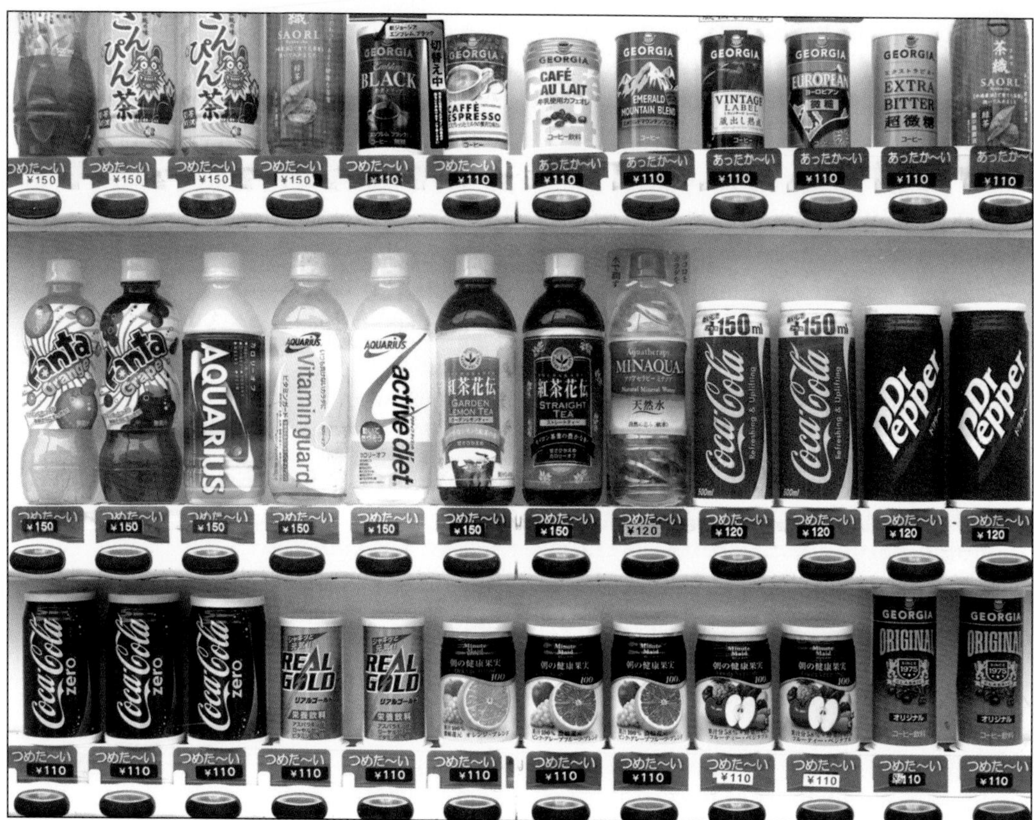

Caffeinated substances, including coffee, tea, sodas, and chocolate, stimulate the nervous system and may contribute to insomnia.

nicotine can contribute to insomnia is by interrupting sleep. Because nicotine is an addictive drug, it is craved by the smoker's body. This craving does not disappear during the night. As smokers sleep, their bodies go through nicotine withdrawal. This may cause them to awaken in the middle of the night.[27]

Diagnosis and Treatment

An individual who suffers from short-term insomnia may be fortunate enough to see it go away on its own after a few days or weeks. Those burdened with chronic insomnia, however, are not so lucky. An undetermined number of these long-term insomniacs end up going to a doctor, hospital, or sleep clinic to seek diagnoses and treatment.

Depending on the circumstances, diagnosing the condition may include a physical exam, a medical history, a sleep history, a sleep study, or some combination of these. In the physical exam, the doctor will try to rule out other medical problems that could be causing the patient's insomnia. To do this thoroughly, it might be necessary for the patient to have a blood test.

If the doctor wants a medical history, he or she will ask whether the patient has been experiencing any ongoing health problems such as depression or arthritis. The doctor will ask whether the person has had any painful injuries recently that might be contributing to the sleep problems. The doctor will likely also ask whether the patient takes any medicines on a regular basis; exercises regularly and if so, in what manner; uses caffeine, tobacco, and/or alcohol; or suffers from unusual amounts of stress.

When a sleep history is called for, the doctor will inquire about how frequently the patient has difficulty sleeping and how long he or she has suffered with the problem. The doctor will also ask whether the patient eats, drinks, or takes any medicines before going to bed and whether there are any distractions in the bedroom, such as a radio, television, or computer. Other typical questions, according to the NHLBI, include:

> When do you go to bed and get up on workdays and days off? How long does it take you to fall asleep? How often do you wake up at night? How long does it take you to fall back asleep? Do you snore loudly and often or wake up gasping or feeling out of breath? How refreshed do you feel when you wake up and how tired do you feel during the day? How often do you doze off or have trouble staying awake during routine tasks, especially driving?[28]

In some cases the doctor may ask the patient to go home and keep a sleep diary for a week or more. Each morning, the person describes in writing what the sleep experience was like during the previous night and how he or she feels that morning. Such a diary might also mention whether and when the patient takes naps and how long they are.

HEALTH FACT

The NIH's MedlinePlus website points out that drinking alcohol or smoking tobacco before bedtime makes the effects of insomnia worse.

In cases where a doctor, clinic, or hospital believes that it is warranted, the patient may also undergo a sleep study, called a polysomnogram. This procedure takes place at a sleep center staffed by medical personnel who specialize in sleep disorders. There the patient goes to sleep, and his or her eye movements, breathing, chest movements, heart rate, brain activity, blood pressure, and blood oxygen content are all monitored and recorded.

Using some or all of these diagnostic processes, a doctor can get a fairly accurate idea of the patient's specific sleep problem and from that prescribe some sort of treatment.

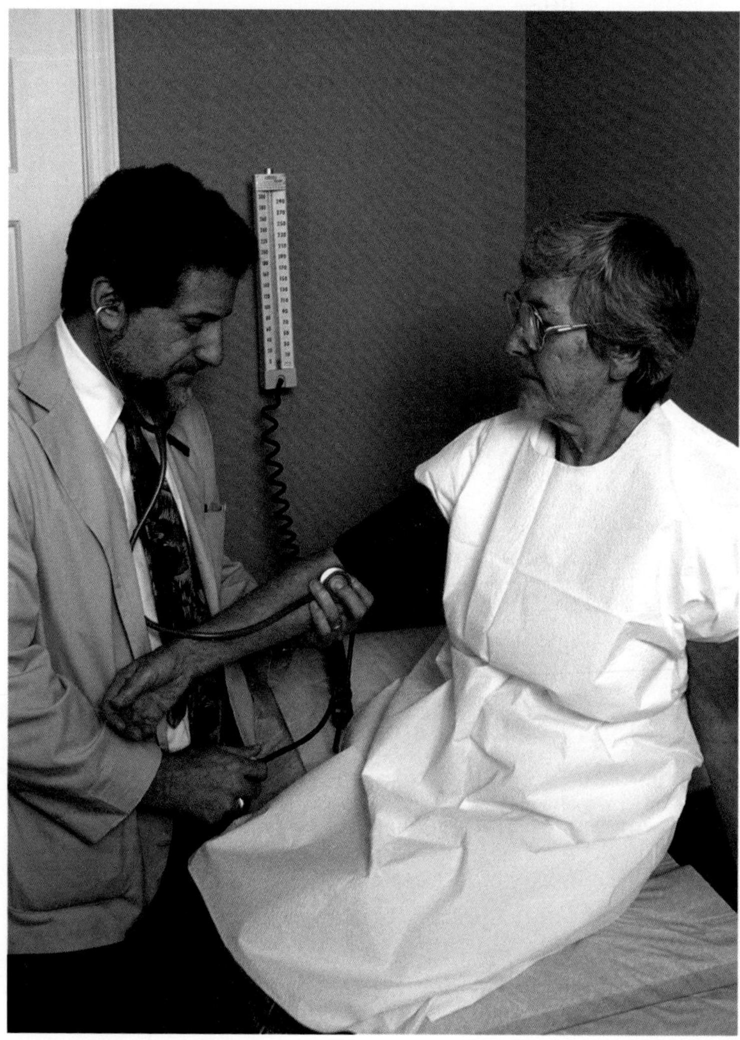

A physical exam, a medical and sleep history, a sleep study, or a combination of all these may be necessary to accurately diagnose insomnia.

Noted sleep specialist Louis R. Chanin provides a brief overview of some of the standard approaches to treating insomnia:

> Mild insomnia often can be prevented or cured by practicing good sleep habits. If your insomnia makes it hard for you to function during the day because you are sleepy and tired, your health care provider may prescribe sleeping pills for a limited time. Rapid onset, short-acting drugs can help you avoid effects such as drowsiness the following day. . . . Treatment for chronic insomnia includes first treating any underlying conditions or health problems that are causing the insomnia. If insomnia continues, your health care provider may suggest behavioral therapy. Behavioral approaches help you to change behaviors that may worsen insomnia and to learn new behaviors to promote sleep.[29]

Not to Be Ignored

Evidence shows that whatever treatment a doctor might recommend, getting a diagnosis by a medical professional is highly advisable for anyone who suffers from chronic insomnia. If for no other reason, it might save the person a good deal of trouble and grief by catching some completely unexpected problem. As medical editor Michelle Andrews says, "There's good reason not to ignore insomnia. It often signals other medical or psychiatric problems, particularly in women, and a savvy practitioner may diagnose and treat an underlying problem that would otherwise escape detection."[30]

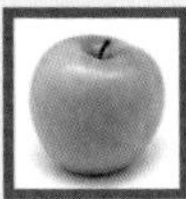

CHAPTER 3

Other Common Sleep Disorders

Although insomnia affects more people by far than any other single sleep disorder, sleep experts say that most of the others need to be taken seriously, too. In all, more than eighty sleep disorders are recognized by the American Academy of Sleep Medicine. (Located in Darien, Illinois, the academy, established in 1975, sets universal standards for sleep disorders and boasts a membership of about ten thousand doctors and fifteen hundred sleep centers.)

Of these numerous sleep problems three of the most widespread and uncomfortable are sleep apnea (or obstructive sleep apnea), restless legs syndrome (RLS), and narcolepsy. Anyone who suffers from these disorders should see a sleep specialist, says Nancy Foldvary-Schaefer. Such conditions can cause a person to lose sleep on a regular basis, she points out, and "a lack of sleep can build up over time, creating a sleep deficit that deprives the body of time necessary to repair and rejuvenate itself. This situation, in turn, can lead to serious complications and health hazards, including high blood pressure, weight gain, anxiety and depression, academic underachievement, poor work performance, and motor vehicle accidents."[31]

The Unrecognized Killer

Such health hazards are often caused by sleep apnea, a very common and potentially life-threatening sleep problem. Defined as simply as possible, *sleep apnea* means that while sleeping a person stops breathing for ten to fifteen or more seconds. This happens not just once but from ten to thirty or more times each hour. It is not unusual for the person to experience such a lapse in breathing up to two hundred times or more in a typical night. Usually, the person resumes normal breathing after several seconds, at times emitting a sharp choking or snorting noise. Yet there is always the

A doctor conducts apnea research. Because sleep apnea is difficult to detect, it is being widely studied.

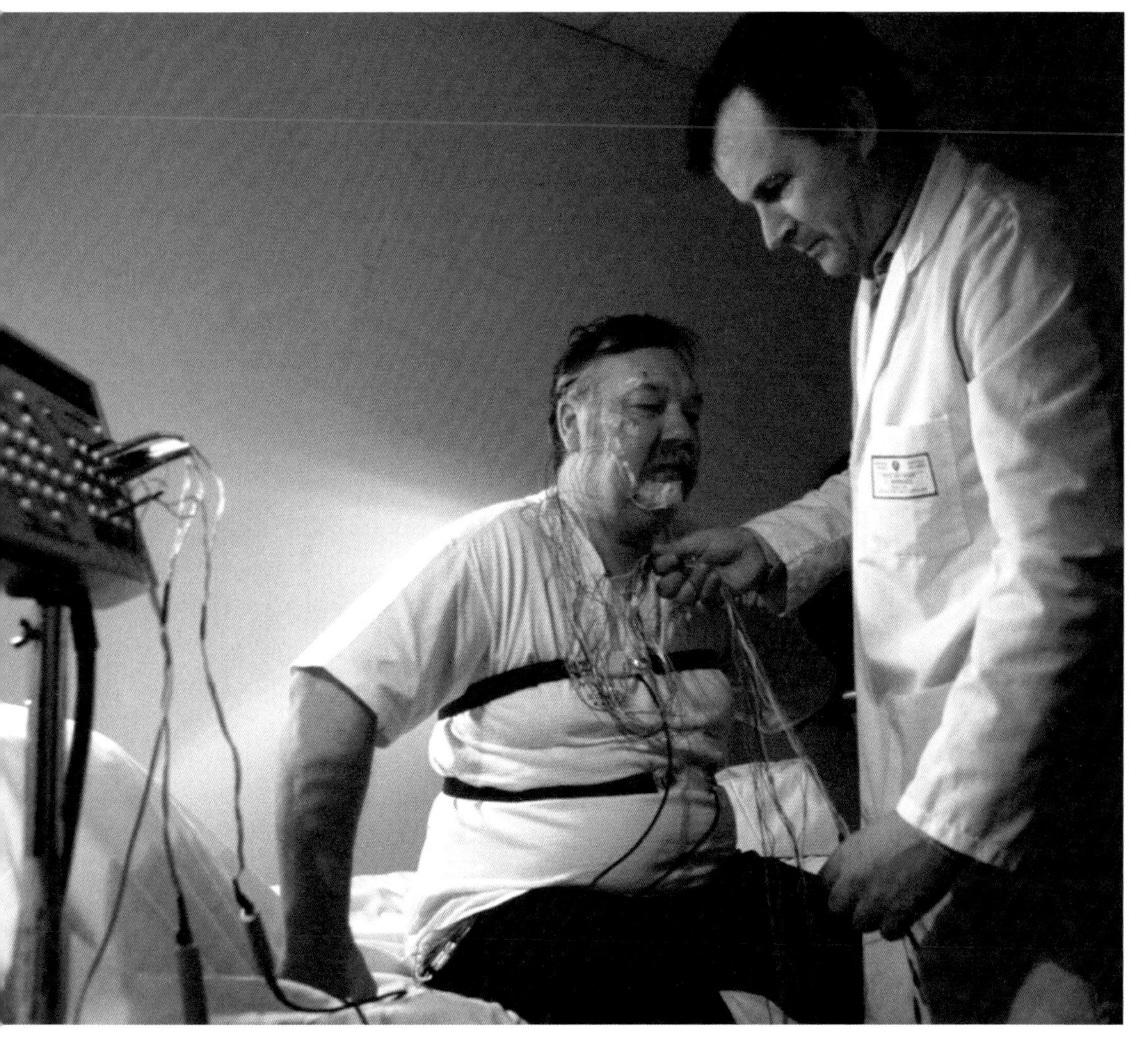

chance that the next breathing lapse will be permanent and result in suffocation and death. In William Dement's words:

> Apnea is an unrecognized killer, but it is hiding in plain sight. Every night more than 50 million Americans stop breathing. In a stunning evolutionary failure, nature endowed us with throats that tend to collapse during sleep and stop air flow but did not endow our sleeping brain with the ability to start breathing again calmly. At this breathless moment, the immediate future holds only two possibilities—death or waking up to breathe. . . . [Yet] just when death seems imminent, the sleeper suddenly struggles awake and the tongue and throat muscles tighten, allowing oxygen to flood into the lungs in a series of gasping, snorting breaths. Oxygen is restored to the blood, and the fatal course is reversed. Instead of being alarmed and staying awake, the victim is immediately asleep again. After a few seconds, snoring begins—and the cycle starts again.[32]

Sleep apnea, with its frightening series of breathing stoppages, is more often than not chronic and significantly reduces the quality of a person's sleep. This makes the person periodically drowsy during the day and thereby more susceptible than average to irritability, poor work performance, and car accidents. Regarding the latter, Carlos H. Schenck states, "Researchers in Virginia compared the driving records of patients with sleep apnea to those without. They discovered that the automobile-accident rate of the patients with sleep apnea was 2.6 times the accident rate of all licensed drivers in the state of Virginia, and that 24 percent of patients with sleep apnea reported falling asleep at least once per week while driving."[33]

In fact, sleep apnea is a chief cause of daytime tiredness, as tens of millions of American adults suffer from the disorder. Dement estimates that up to 20 percent of the adult population, or more than 60 million people, have it. Experts say that children get it, too, but for technical reasons, determining their numbers is more difficult than it is for adults; rough estimates range from as low as 2 percent to as high as 20 percent. Even in adults, the condition can often be hard to identify. According to the NHLBI, "Sleep apnea often goes undiagnosed. Doctors usually can't detect the condition during routine office visits. Also, no blood test can help diagnose the condition. Most people who have sleep apnea don't know they have it because it only occurs during sleep. A family member or bed partner might be the first to notice signs of sleep apnea."[34]

Although difficult to detect in specific individuals, sleep apnea has been widely studied by the medical community, which has learned who is most at risk for it. The disorder occurs more or less equally among men and woman, but the risk of developing it increases among people who are overweight,

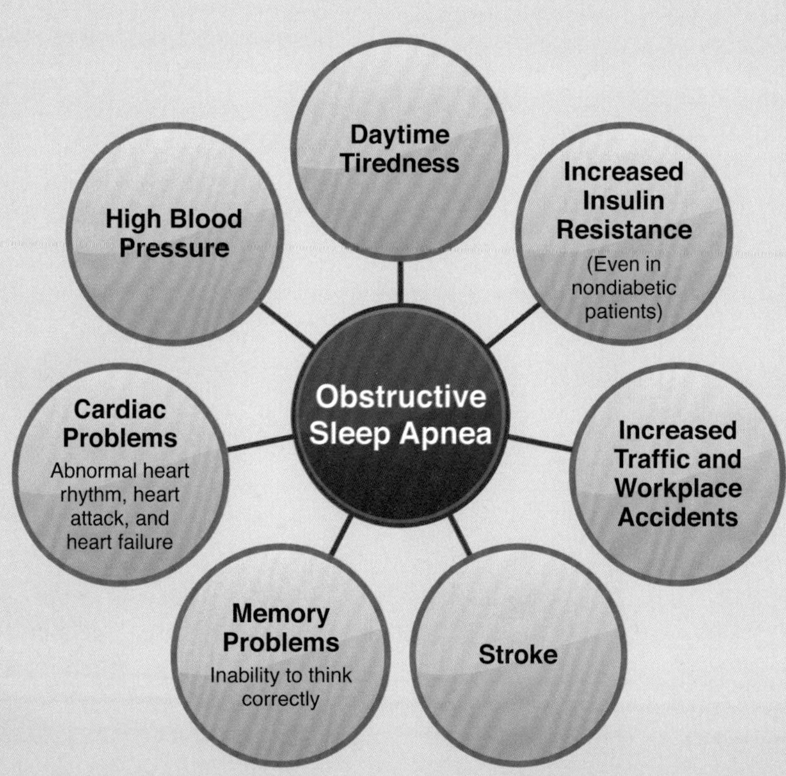

Taken from: Denton Sleep Disorders Center. www.dentonsleepdisorderlab.com/obstructive-sleep-apnea.html.

especially those who are obese. People who have a smaller-than-average upper airway or a larger-than-average tongue that partially blocks their airway are also more at risk. In addition, having a small jaw, a bigger-than-average overbite, and/or a larger-than-average neck circumference can raise a person's risk

Sleep Apnea and Overweight People

One of the many facts that came out of sleep research in the last few decades is that the severity of sleep apnea is directly related to a person's weight, as explained here by noted sleep expert Carlos H. Schenck. He uses the measure known as body mass index, or BMI, which estimates a person's body fat based on his or her weight and height. A BMI of roughly 19 to 25 is considered normal, and a BMI of 30 or above is seen as obese.

> In a population-based study of 6,132 participants 40 years old or older, researchers determined that the more severe sleep apnea is, the more likely it is that the sufferer is obese. Among those with mild sleep apnea, 16.4 percent had a normal body mass index (less than 25), 38.1 percent were overweight (BMI of 25 to less than 30), and 45.5 percent were obese (BMI of 30 or more). Among those with moderate sleep apnea, 13.9 percent had a normal BMI, 32.6 percent were overweight, and 53.5 percent were obese. Among those with severe sleep apnea, 10.2 percent had a normal BMI, 28.7 percent were overweight, and 61.1 percent were obese.

Carlos H. Schenck. *Sleep.* New York: Avery, 2008, pp. 34–35.

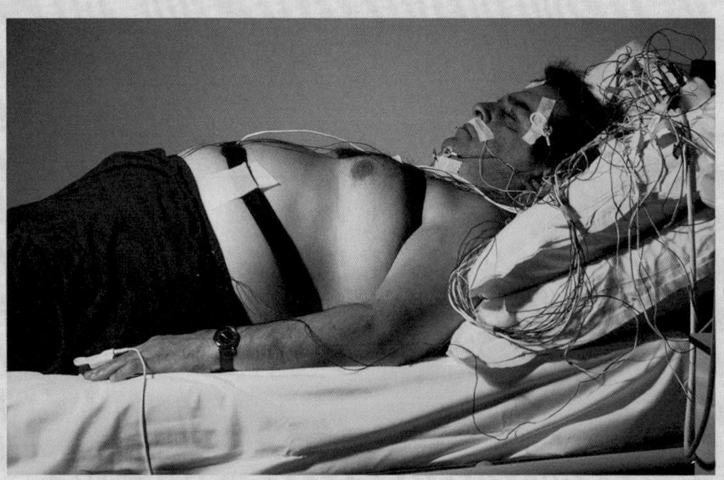

Research shows that obese people are more likely to have sleep apnea.

of developing sleep apnea. Smoking and drinking alcohol both increase the risk as well. Finally, for reasons that are unclear, the risk of developing the condition is higher among certain ethnic groups, including Hispanics, African Americans, and Pacific Islanders.

Symptoms and Treatment

By doing sleep studies, in which patients are observed sleeping through the night in the controlled setting of a sleep center, sleep detectives have compiled a reliable list of symptoms for this debilitating condition. First and foremost on the list is repeated, often noisy snoring. Not all snoring is related to sleep apnea, the experts caution, but a large proportion of people who chronically snore *do* have the disorder. In fact, sleep apnea and snoring often go together like a pair of tag-team wrestlers, as noted by Dement, who morbidly but quite aptly calls them "the midnight stranglers." He provides one of the clearest available descriptions of what happens during snoring: "The throat's rigidity for breathing is accompanied partly with the help of muscular tension. But when we go to sleep, suction and air passing through the throat cause its soft sides to pull inward. As the throat is pulled inward, rebounds, and pulls inward again, it sets up a rapid vibration, like a flag rippling on a windy day. The vibrating flesh creates a loud rumble—snoring."[35]

When someone snores loudly, his or her breathing is strained, Dement explains, and his or her throat nearly closes up. The tighter and more restricted the throat becomes when the person inhales, the harder it becomes for the diaphragm to heave and draw enough air for normal breathing. The result, according to Dement, "is a vicious cycle in which increasing suction from the lungs and increasing air flow through the throat pull the throat closed even more, making the vibration stronger, and the snoring louder."[36] Thus, in people whose throats are narrow and therefore susceptible to sleep apnea, snoring signals the approach of the long pause in breathing that characterizes the disorder.

Other symptoms of sleep apnea are the frequent pauses in breathing themselves, gasping for air and/or choking while asleep, feeling tired after waking up, and experiencing periods of grogginess during the rest of the day. It is also common for people with sleep apnea to have periodic bouts with chest pain, shortness of breath, dry throat, headaches, and/or nasal congestion. Still other, though less common, symptoms are sexual dysfunction and learning and memory difficulties.

Once it has been diagnosed, treatments for severe sleep apnea usually begin with the patient's use of a continuous positive airway pressure device (CPAP). It consists of a sort of mask that fits over the nose or nose and mouth and helps keep the throat open during sleep. Studies have shown that if a CPAP is used faithfully every night, in most cases the apnea stops or at least is significantly reduced. If this approach does not work, doctors might recommend a dental appliance that changes the position of the tongue and jaw or surgery to remove the excess tissue that is blocking the airway. Lifestyle changes can also be effective—among them losing weight if one is obese, quitting smoking, and avoiding alcoholic beverages.

A man uses a continuous positive airway pressure (CPAP) device to treat his sleep apnea. If used every night, such devices can significantly reduce the incidence of sleep apnea.

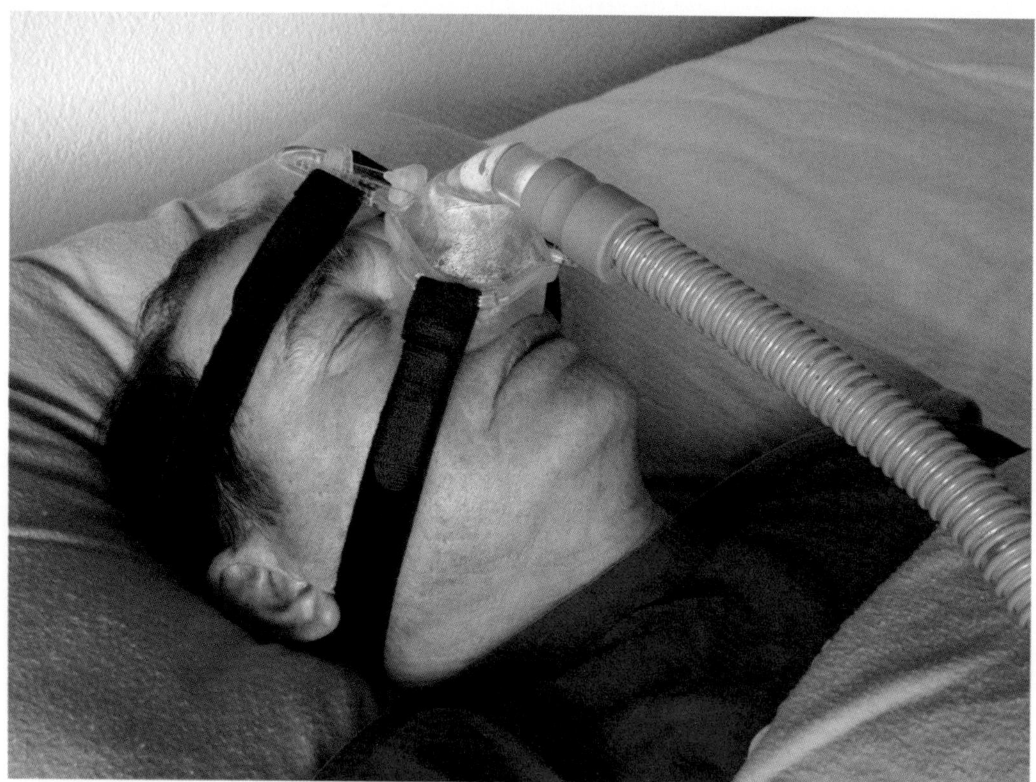

Restless Legs Syndrome (RLS)

Unlike sleep apnea, which is mostly about breathing, another common sleep disorder—RLS (also known as Willis-Ekbom disease)—is mostly about sensations felt in the legs. As Max Hirshkowitz explains, "People with RLS experience unusual, crawling sensations in their legs (usually their calves). RLS sufferers move their legs constantly, seeking relief from the strange feelings. For people with severe RLS, the urge to move their legs is almost irresistible because moving *does* relieve their discomfort, however briefly."[37]

At first glance, such descriptions may make it appear that the discomfort involved is minor and that the disorder itself is fairly trivial compared with other sleep disorders. This impression is mistaken, however. People with moderate to severe cases of RLS often find it difficult to fall asleep, and/or they wake up several times during the night. For this reason, RLS is sometimes the root cause of secondary insomnia, which makes a person feel sleepy during the daytime. Thus, RLS can ultimately cause poor performance at work or in school, as well as car accidents, sleep experts say, and therefore needs to be taken seriously.

According to the National Sleep Foundation, RLS affects about 10 percent of American adults. A 2005 study involving sixteen thousand people in the United States and five European countries found that roughly 5 percent of the adult population experience RLS symptoms at least once a week. Another 3 percent of adults have symptoms twice a week or more. Also, a recent study of ten thousand families in the United States and United Kingdom showed that around 2 percent of children experience RLS on a regular basis. (In the past, many children displaying RLS symptoms were erroneously diagnosed with "growing pains," now known to be a fictitious condition.) In addition, various studies have demonstrated that women are 50 percent more likely to be bothered by RLS than are men.

Another important fact revealed by recent research is that RLS is often misdiagnosed as other disorders or physical problems. These include insomnia,

HEALTH FACT

According to the CDC, RLS may be at least partially caused by abnormal amounts (too little or too much) of a substance called dopamine in a person's body.

muscular and orthopedic conditions, and depression. The Restless Legs Syndrome Foundation (or RLS Foundation, founded in 1992 in Rochester, Minnesota) says that about 40 percent of people with RLS report having symptoms identical to those of depression. This explains why some doctors and other medical authorities mistakenly diagnose those with RLS as having depression.

RLS's Causes and Treatment

As for what causes RLS, to date no one has been able to say for sure. Following is the RLS Foundation's official statement on RLS's causes and connections to other medical conditions:

> Extensive research into the cause of RLS is occurring worldwide. A single unifying cause has not been identified, but we are getting closer. Here is what we do know. First, RLS often runs in families. This is called primary or familial RLS. Researchers are currently looking for the gene or genes that cause RLS. The disorder sometimes appears to be a result of another condition, which, when present, worsens the underlying RLS. This is called secondary RLS. Up to 25 percent of women develop RLS during pregnancy but symptoms often disappear after giving birth. Anemia and low iron levels frequently contribute to a worsening of RLS. In addition, RLS is very common in patients requiring dialysis for end-stage renal disease.[38]

The RLS Foundation has also called attention to recent studies conducted by Johns Hopkins University and Pennsylvania State University. Their research has uncovered some evidence indicating that RLS might be caused by a deficiency, or lack, of iron in the brain. At first, the researchers examined fluid from the spine. Then they performed autopsies (post-death dissections) of the brains of people who had been diagnosed with RLS. These studies suggest that people with RLS may have trouble distributing the iron they get from food to all parts of the body. If that is indeed the case, it means on the one hand that RLS is not caused by brain damage, as had been suspected. On the other hand, the studies hint that finding a

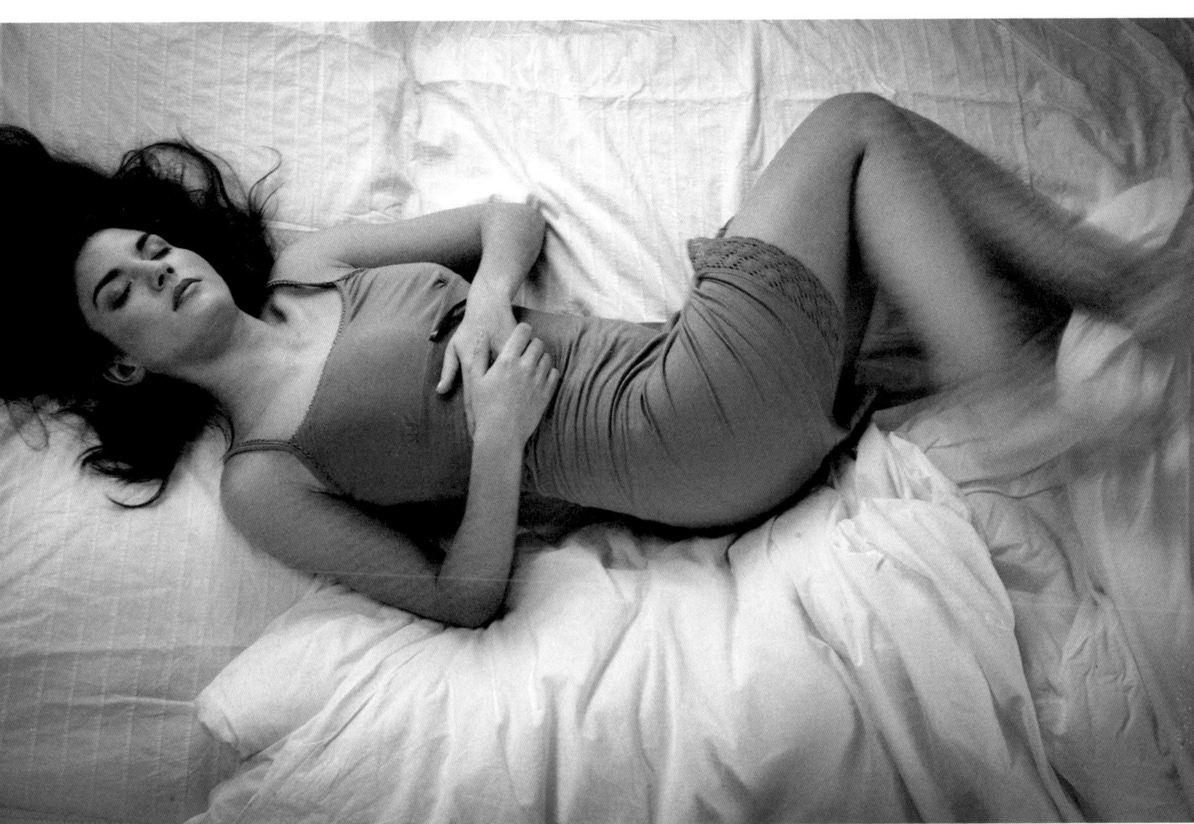

way for people with RLS to better regulate the iron in their system might lead to an effective treatment for the disorder.

People with restless legs syndrome experience crawling or tingling sensations in their legs, which causes twitching and interferes with sleep.

Unfortunately for those with RLS, until recently no medicines approved by the U.S. Food and Drug Administration to treat the disorder existed. In 2006 a drug called Mirapex was approved for treating moderate and severe RLS. In clinical trials, Mirapex relieved the odd sensations in the legs of those with RLS and thereby helped these people sleep better and have a better quality of life.

The drug does produce several side effects, however—among them dizziness and nausea. More recently, researchers showed that treating RLS patients with some medicines approved for other conditions temporarily reduces the classic symptoms of RLS. In addition, people with severe RLS have found some relief by engaging in physical activities such as walking, stretching, rubbing the legs, applying hot and cold packs to the legs, and practicing yoga.

RLS and PLMS at the Same Time

Harvard University's Lawrence J. Epstein cites the case of a fifty-seven-year-old schoolteacher named Maria who suffered from two similar sleep disorders at the same time—RLS and periodic limb movements disorder (PLMS). PLMS is characterized by repetitive twitches in the lower limbs that happen about every twenty to forty seconds during sleep. This case study demonstrates that such disorders are easily treatable.

> When she came to see me, she said she was so tired she rarely left the house. In fact, that morning she hadn't had enough energy to get dressed and arrived in her nightgown and robe, with rollers still in her hair. A sleep study showed that severe periodic limb movement disorder was disturbing her sleep in addition to the RLS she experienced while awake. I started her on a dopamine agent [a medicine often used to treat sleep disorders] to treat both. When Maria returned a month later, she was a changed woman. She was well-dressed [and] wide awake. She said her leg discomfort was gone, she slept great at night, and she was no longer sleepy all day.

Lawrence J. Epstein. *The Harvard Medical School Guide to a Good Night's Sleep.* New York: McGraw-Hill, 2007, p. 146.

Medical experts say that these approaches to alleviating the vexing symptoms of RLS should be supplemented by certain coping techniques. First, they say, those with RLS should not hide their symptoms, but rather should be open about the condition with family, friends, and coworkers. Such people are likely to sympathize with individuals who have RLS and become their support group. Second, those with RLS should arrange their daily schedule so that they sleep when the unpleasant leg sensations are least prominent. They should also select an aisle seat in airplanes and at the movies. That will allow them to stretch their legs or get up for a short walk if the symptoms become too bothersome.

Narcolepsy: "The Yin to Insomnia's Yang"

RLS has something fundamentally in common with sleep apnea and insomnia—namely that in all three disorders, an individual has difficulty falling asleep. The case is very different with another serious sleep problem—narcolepsy. Narcoleptics actually fall asleep too easily. According to Harvard University researcher Lawrence J. Epstein:

> Narcolepsy is a debilitating disorder in which people experience overwhelming waves of drowsiness that may strike at any hour of the day, putting them to sleep during conversations, meetings, meals, and other ordinary activities. In this respect, narcolepsy can be considered the opposite of insomnia—the yin to insomnia's yang—since an insomniac has trouble falling asleep and a narcoleptic has trouble staying awake.[39]

Narcolepsy is a sleep disorder that causes people to suddenly fall asleep during normal everyday activities.

Another important fact about narcoleptics is that the common perception they are almost always sleepy is incorrect. In fact, as a rule they sleep about as much as an average person does. The central problem for those with narcolepsy is that they have difficulty controlling *when* they sleep. Narcoleptics may have what they feel is a good night's

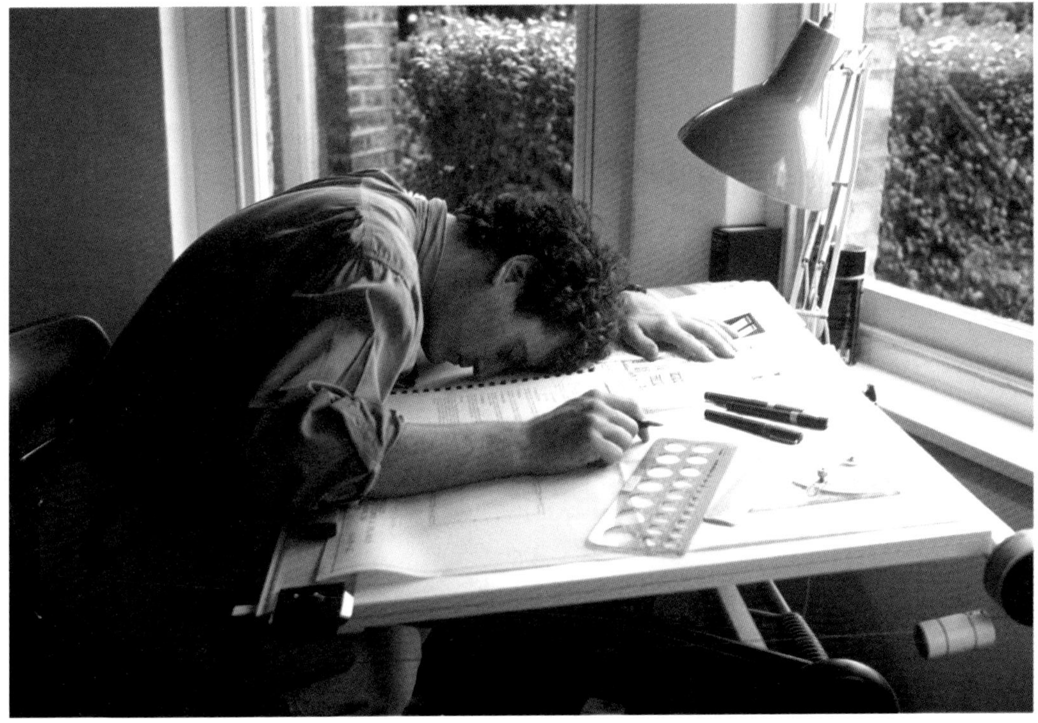

sleep, get up, get dressed, and go to work feeling perfectly fine. Then, in the middle of the afternoon, perhaps while sitting with coworkers at lunch or in a meeting, they suddenly drop off to sleep. One expert observer calls such an episode a "sleep attack."[40] Research shows that the disorder can afflict both genders equally, typically starts in adolescence, and usually gets more pronounced as people age. Often, narcoleptics suffer with the disorder for a long time without seeing a doctor, mainly because they do not realize they have a medical condition. Many narcoleptics later say that they thought their odd sleep episodes happened simply because their bodies needed the sleep.

Symptoms That Can Be Frightening

Besides sudden drowsiness, narcolepsy has other symptoms or variations. Individuals may see or hear things that are not actually there right before nodding off. Also, without warning they may feel weak and lose control of most or all of their muscles, a state called cataplexy. This occurs more often than not when narcoleptics are upset, excited, very surprised, or feeling some other strong emotion. Narcoleptics may experience a feeling of paralysis as well, making them incapable of moving just before falling asleep or just after waking up. In addition, people who have narcolepsy tend to start dreaming immediately after going to sleep.

This last symptom, immediate dreaming, is a clue to what is occurring internally during a narcoleptic sleep episode and, in turn, the cause of the condition. In normal sleep a person goes through a series of stages—from stage one to stages two, three, and four of non-REM sleep, and finally to REM sleep. It usually takes an hour and sometimes up to an hour and a half to reach the REM sleep stage. Experts say that this cycle of sleep stages depends to some degree on the brain's normal production of a chemical known as hypocretin. The problem for narcoleptics is that their brain does not produce enough of this substance. As a result, the National Sleep Foundation explains, their sleep episode "begins almost immediately with REM sleep and fragments of REM occur involuntarily throughout the

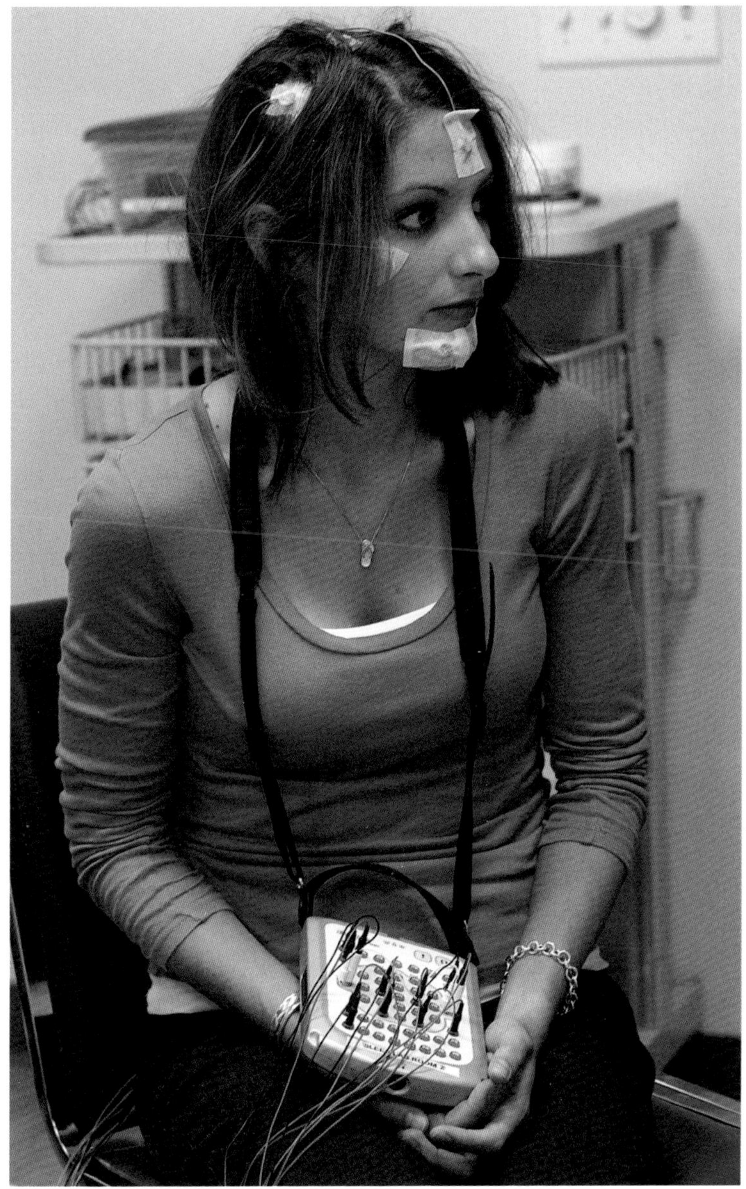

Sensors attached to this narcolepsy patient's head monitor REM sleep patterns. Narcolepsy symptoms are often frightening for the sufferer.

waking hours. When you consider that during REM sleep our muscles are paralyzed and dreaming occurs, it is not surprising that narcolepsy is associated with paralysis, hallucinations, and other dream-like and dramatically debilitating symptoms."[41]

Some of these extra symptoms, or in a sense digressions, that a narcoleptic can experience can be frightening, even

HEALTH FACT

Some narcoleptics display a bizarre symptom called microsleep, according to the National Sleep Foundation. During the daytime, they experience an extremely brief sleep episode lasting a second or two and then go on working, talking, or doing other activities without even realizing what happened.

if they do not always result in injury. Cataplexy—loss of muscle control—for example, can be scary because it makes a person feel helpless. In some cases the person actually collapses onto the floor or ground. Fortunately for these individuals, as Epstein points out, the onset of such an episode is not instantaneous. "These falls occur slowly," he says. "So they rarely cause injuries," because the narcoleptic can feel the attack approaching and goes into what might be called a controlled fall. "The person is usually fully awake," Epstein adds, "and aware of what's going on, but is unable to talk and *appears* to be asleep. Although cataplexy sometimes leads to sleep, usually the person recovers spontaneously after several seconds or minutes."[42]

Similarly, sleep paralysis, which 50 to 60 percent of narcoleptics suffer from, can be terrifying the first few times a person experiences it. As described by those who have gone through it, one is gripped by a dread that breathing will no longer be possible. Also, REM sleep starts to take hold, causing the onset of fleeting hallucinations. As with cataplexy, however, individuals frequently become accustomed to such attacks. They learn that in reality, as Epstein says, "breathing is not affected, so these episodes are less alarming in subsequent occurrences."[43]

"No Picnic!"

No cure currently exists for narcolepsy. Two treatments, which help some individuals more than others, are behavioral therapies and medications that help regulate sleep. In the behavioral approach, narcoleptics may take three or more planned naps during the day in hopes of lessening the chances of unwanted episodes. They also avoid heavy meals and alcohol, both of which tend to cause drowsiness.

Yet the fact that many narcoleptics learn to avoid or control some of their sleep attacks should not detract from the seriousness of the disorder. With extremely rare exceptions, it is permanent. Moreover, narcoleptics are highly susceptible to developing other sleep disorders, including sleep apnea, as they age. In the words of a longtime narcoleptic who prefers to remain anonymous:

> Sure, I can control it fairly well most of the time. But you never know when it's going to hit and whether it's this time that you'll finally fall the wrong way and crack your head open. You also never know who's going to be watching you when it hits. Some people just don't understand. You know what I mean? They never treat you the same again. Take it from me. Having to live with a sleep disorder is no picnic![44]

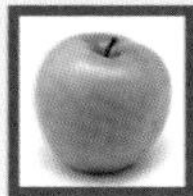

CHAPTER **4**

Weird Behaviors While Sleeping

Quite a number of sleep disorders fall into a category of related conditions that sleep scientists call parasomnias. (When combined, the Greek prefix *para* and the Latin term *somnus* become *parasomnia*, meaning "faulty sleep.") They are behaviors that are seen as normal (though not necessarily desirable or acceptable) when enacted while awake, but are viewed as decidedly *abnormal* and/or weird when someone does them while asleep.

Among the best-known or more familiar examples of parasomnias are sleepwalking and bed-wetting. Walking and urinating are obviously perfectly normal acts when performed by someone who is awake and aware. However, walking or urinating in one's sleep are behaviors to be avoided if possible. Less familiar to most people are parasomnias such as sleep talking, sleep terrors (episodes of extreme fear while asleep), eating while asleep, and REM sleep behavior disorder (acting violently while asleep). Some people even engage in sexual relations, sometimes called "sleepsex," while sleeping.

Parasomnias are far from rare; experts estimate that an average of about 10 percent of Americans, or more than 30 million people in the United States, suffer from one kind or another. Parasomnias can affect people of any age. But these disorders tend to be more common in children. Up to 30 percent of children sleepwalk at least on occasion, for instance, but only about 5 percent or so of adults sleepwalk. Fortunately for them, the other 25 percent of young sleepwalkers eventually outgrow it.

Medical authorities are not completely certain what causes most parasomnias. But increasing numbers of sleep

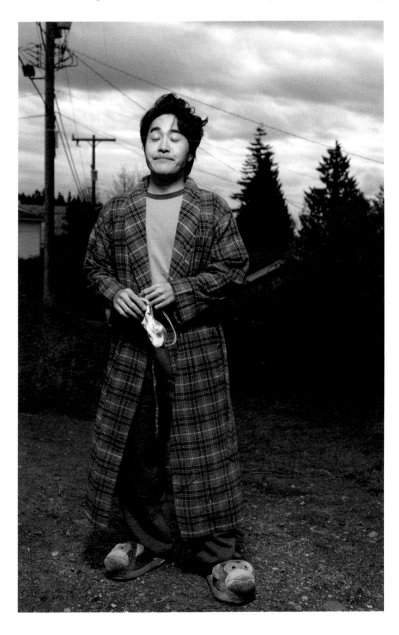

The best-known example of parasomnia is sleepwalking.

specialists are leaning toward accepting a theory for which Max Hirshkowitz provides this concise overview:

> Sleep states overlap during the transition from one stage of sleep to another. But these transitions are usually smooth and of no consequence to the sleeper. But in people with parasomnias, something goes amiss with the sequencing of their sleep-wake cycle. Part of their brain is aroused and may be partially awake while another part is diving into the cool, inviting depths of deeper sleep. This lack of synchronization [smooth timing] produces odd physical behaviors, usually because they're behaviors people associate with wakefulness, and yet, people with certain parasomnias can be exceedingly difficult to arouse to complete awareness. If you do manage to wake them up, they're likely to be confused, afraid, or combative. They're still in that twilight world, not yet fully awake and yet, not really asleep either.[45]

Sleepwalking Episodes

One of the most prominent residents of that strange twilight world is the sleepwalker. The technical name for sleepwalking is somnambulism (and a sleepwalker is a somnambulist). It consists not only of walking around, but also of performing other, at times complex behaviors while sleeping. Children sleepwalk much more often than adults do, particularly children aged three to seven. Also, young people who have sleep apnea and/or who wet the bed are more apt to sleepwalk. Among adults, meanwhile, those who are sleep deficient are more likely to walk and do other things in their sleep than are people who get their required amount of sleep.

No matter how involved the physical behaviors of sleepwalkers may be or how much energy they exert, they are in a deep sleep throughout. For that

HEALTH FACT

Max Hirshkowitz and other sleep experts say that parasomnias such as sleepwalking and sleep talking tend to run in families; many of the people with these disorders may carry genetic factors that make suffering from them more likely.

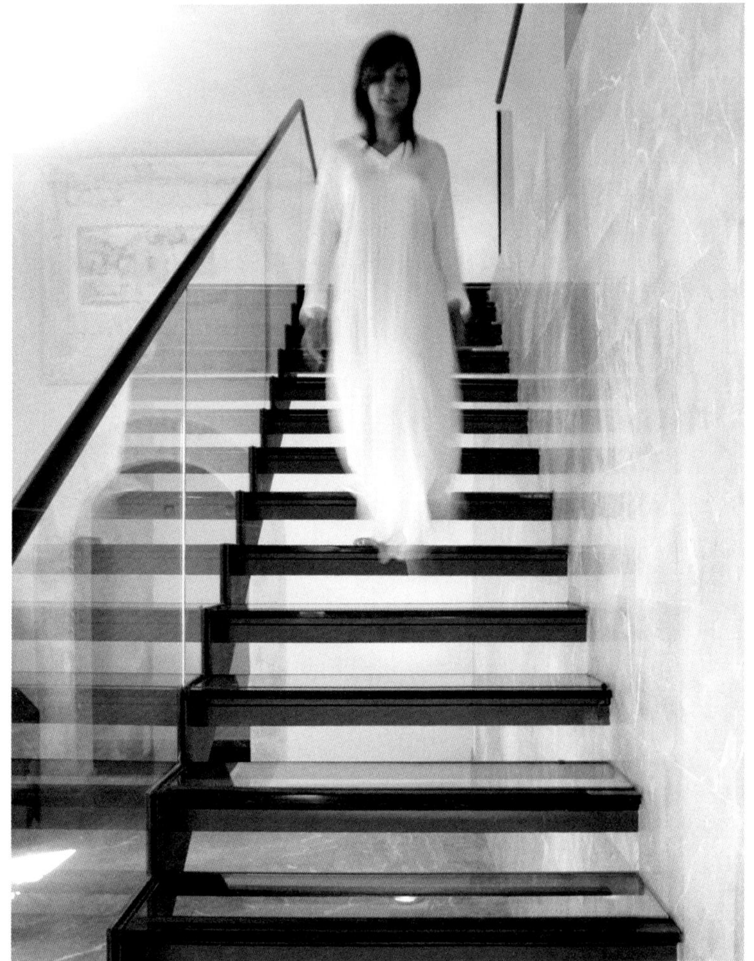

Sleepwalkers are difficult to waken and can exhibit other behaviors while sleepwalking, such as talking, using foul language, exhibiting poor physical coordination, and urinating in inappropriate places.

reason, they are usually very hard to wake up. (The notion that it is dangerous to wake up a sleepwalker is a myth.) Moreover, it is unlikely they will remember the sleepwalking episode. When sleepwalkers do finally awaken, they are more often than not confused, and if someone points out the episode they may even refuse to believe it occurred. It is also important to point out that sleepwalkers are *not* acting out their dreams, as is commonly supposed. In fact, sleepwalking episodes happen in non-REM sleep, when no dreaming is going on.

In addition to doing various physical activities while asleep and being hard to wake up, sleepwalkers exhibit several other symptoms, which differ slightly in number and

The Sleep-Talking Couple

A widely respected sleep specialist told the story of a married couple who came to see him because of what they viewed as a bizarre and embarrassing problem they were having in bed at night. He diagnosed them both as classic sleep talkers and later described their case, saying in part:

> One night the wife sat up [and] began sleep-talking. This triggered a confusional arousal [awakening in a state of confusion] in her husband, who also sat up and began talking. The two of them were bewildered and feeding off each other, having a strange conversation that escalated in complexity—and eventually they began shouting at each other. They lived in an apartment complex, and the neighbors woke up and were about to call the police. A neighbor came over and banged on the couple's door, which caused one of them to snap out of the confusional arousal and answer the door. Both of them were horrified. They had no idea they'd been talking, much less shouting, in the middle of the night. And they were very thankful that the police hadn't been called yet. . . . That's what brought them to see me. They were very worried that the next episode would result in a police visit.

Carlos H. Schenck. *Sleep*. New York: Avery, 2008, pp. 235–236.

kind from person to person. Some sleepwalkers talk during an episode, for example, although their words are typically not rational. Doing inappropriate things, like urinating on the floor or using foul language, is also common. Other symptoms include having the eyes open despite being asleep, mumbling incoherently, and displaying poor judgment and coordination.

When sleepwalkers find out that they have displayed such behaviors, they are usually sorry for any inconvenience they may have caused others. It is also common for sleepwalkers to be afraid of what might happen when they are both sleeping and awake. This was demonstrated in a case study cited by Carlos H. Schenck. A patient named Jan came to see him and told him she had been sleepwalking all her life. She said that sometimes incidents—including some in which she hallucinated the presence of a nonexistent visitor—that happened during the short wakeful periods of a typical night frightened her. "There were many times," she explained, that

> I'd wake up in different parts of the house. Sometimes I would be totally naked and not know why. And when I looked down the stairs to figure out where I was, there was an image of a shadow in the doorway or window, and I thought it was a man who was out trying to catch me, and I saw his shadow in the second-floor window, too, so I just felt kind of imprisoned until I could slide down the steps to go to my room. . . . Of course, I was always exhausted in the morning. I felt like I'd been run over by a Mack truck.[46]

Attempts at Treatment

Unfortunately for sleepwalkers, no cure exists for their ailment, nor is there any single universal treatment for it. Instead, doctors have employed a number of different approaches to treatment, some of which have helped with individual patients but do little or nothing for others. Improving sleep hygiene is one common medical recommendation. (Sleep hygiene consists of practices that promote restful sleep, including having a regular bedtime, not eating or drinking alcohol before going to bed, maintaining good nutrition, exercising regularly, and so forth.) Another treatment approach is hypnosis. In addition, some sleep specialists prescribe various medicines, among them drugs that have sedative or hypnotic properties, and/or antidepressants (drugs used to treat depression).

One drug that has shown promise in treating sleepwalking is clonazepam, which has sedative and hypnotic effects in patients. Among other sleep experts, Schenck has had some success with it, including in the case of his patient Jan. He later recalled:

> Jan responded promptly and very well to bedtime clonazepam therapy, and she noticed that not only did it completely stop her sleepwalking, but it also resulted in her feeling much more rested in the morning and throughout the day, allowing her to accomplish more in her life and to feel better all around. For twelve years now, it has kept her disorder under control, and she has not needed to increase the dose of the clonazepam. . . . I have only needed to see Jan for yearly checkup visits, at which time I go over her sleep, the clonazepam therapy, any medical update . . . and [have] an overall discussion about her life and any issues that I should be aware of.[47]

It is important to note that Jan still had occasional minor symptoms of her disorder and that her sleepwalking was not cured. She and Schenck agreed they would adopt the approach of controlling the condition as much as possible using medication. Trying to rid her of the disorder entirely was and remains unfeasible.

Spouting Sleep Speech

Sleepwalkers sometimes engage in another sleep disorder that a fair number of people suffer from separately—sleep talking, technically known as somniloquy (literally meaning "sleep speech"). As its name suggests, it is characterized mainly by talking while asleep, words the sleeper usually does not remember having said after waking up. A few of those words might make sense. But for the most part, sleep speech consists of mumbling, gibberish, and other unintelligible sayings.

Spouting sleep speech affects both children and adults but is far more prevalent in children. Experts estimate that up to 50 percent of children may sleep talk, even if only occasionally and in brief episodes, whereas no more than 5 percent of adults (more men than women) display the disorder.

Other symptoms they may have besides the sleep speech itself are sleepwalking, episodes of sleep apnea, displaying anger or physical violence while asleep, psychiatric problems, and/or seizures similar to those suffered by epileptics.

Sleep specialists say that no specific treatment is necessary for most sleep talkers, especially when they are young, because a majority of them eventually grow out of it. Still, those who do not outgrow it and who suffer with it on a persistent basis should seek medical help. A doctor will look for an underlying cause for the disorder—such as stress, anxiety, or another sleep disorder—and treat that cause accordingly.

HEALTH FACT

When there is a child in the home who sleepwalks, the National Sleep Foundation recommends making sure he or she remains safe by removing breakable or sharp objects from the bedroom, installing gates on stairways, and locking the doors and windows.

Teeth Grinding and Bed-Wetting

Almost as common as sleep talking is another familiar sleep disorder popularly known as teeth grinding. Sleep experts call it bruxism. Those experts think that a majority of people will clench and maybe grind their teeth during sleep on an occasional basis, which is considered normal behavior. If the grinding happens on a regular basis for extended periods, however, the individual likely has the disorder. About 15 percent of children and 5 percent of adults have it and find that it negatively affects their lives. This is because it tends to severely damage the teeth, as well as cause jaw discomfort and other complications.

The exact cause or causes of bruxism are unclear. But most experts have zeroed in on a likely reason for the disorder, described here by Herbert Ross. "Many people believe teeth-grinding serves as an outlet for releasing stress experienced during the day. However, doctors contend that bruxism is the body's way of trying to correct structural problems in the mouth. Nocturnal chewing action may be an attempt to grind upper and lower teeth for a better fit."[48]

The good news for teeth grinders is that the disorder can be treated easily and usually quite effectively. Doctors, most often dentists or dental surgeons, prescribe a mouth guard that fits over the teeth and keeps them from rubbing against each other. The person with the disorder may supplement such a mechanical device with behavioral therapy that includes cutting back on or avoiding caffeine and alcohol consumption. (Evidence indicates that those substances can stimulate teeth-grinding episodes.)

Another familiar parasomnia that affects children more often than adults is nocturnal enuresis, more commonly known as bed-wetting. Most children wet the bed now and then during potty training and occasionally in the years immediately following it, all viewed as normal behavior. But when children continue to wet the bed after the age of six or seven, they may suffer from nocturnal enuresis and need to see a doctor. Ross estimates that up to 3 percent of young people between the ages of twelve and eighteen wet their beds at least sometimes, and a few of them continue doing so as adults.

A common parasomnia problem that affects children is nocturnal enuresis, more commonly known as bed-wetting.

One of the causes of bed-wetting is difficulties with bladder control, which may itself on occasion be a sign of physical abnormalities or damage to the spinal cord, brain, and/or

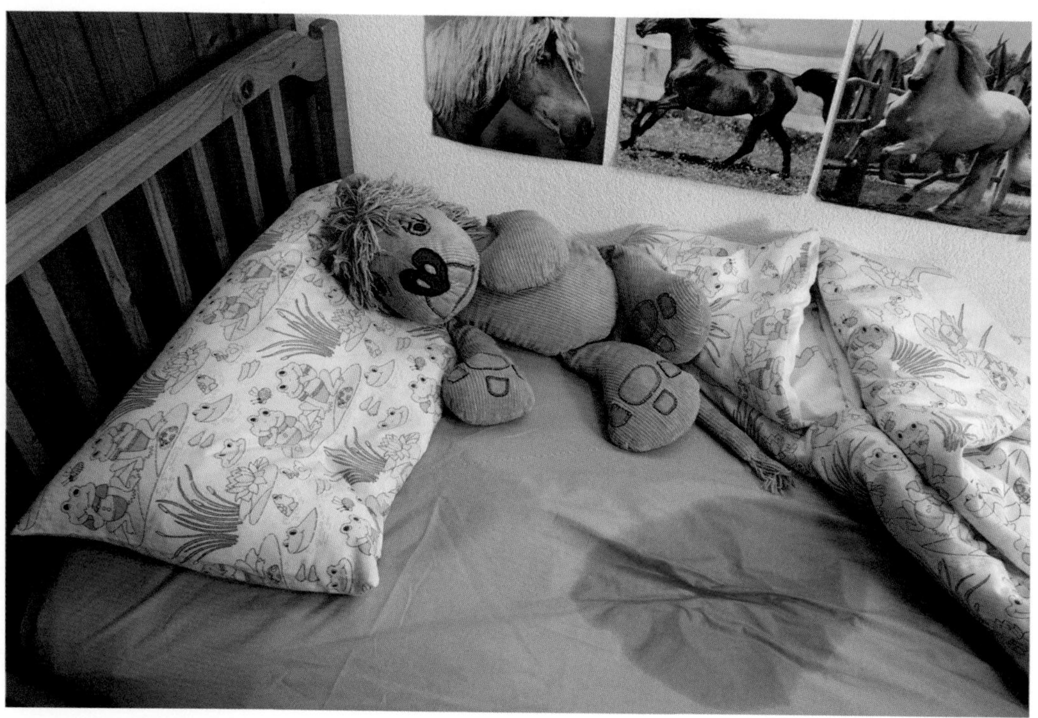

muscles and nerves surrounding the bladder. Or there may be an obstruction of the urinary tract. Much more often, though, according to the experts, the disorder is brought on by stress or some other psychological problem.

Doctors have established some common, simple treatments for bed-wetting. One is to ensure that the affected person goes to the bathroom right before bed each night. Parents of bed wetters should wake them up once or twice during the night and take them to the bathroom. Adults with the disorder should set their alarm clock for periodic bathroom breaks. Also, people of all ages who wet the bed should avoid drinking water or other liquids in the evening after dinner. In addition, in a severe case a doctor may prescribe medication that either relaxes the bladder or works to reduce urine production at night.

Sleep Terrors

Still another example of a sleep disorder that is found more often in children than in adults is the parasomnia best known as sleep terrors (or night terrors). According to Nancy Foldvary-Schaefer:

> Sleep terrors are most common in children between the ages of 3 and 12, and they tend to resolve [go away] during adolescence. As many as 6 percent of children may experience sleep terrors. A much smaller proportion of adults—closer to 2 or 3 percent—experience this disorder. If they occur in adulthood, incidents are most common between the ages of 20 and 30. Few individuals over age 65 experience sleep terrors. Family history may play a strong role in whether your child will experience these episodes.[49]

Most often, such episodes consist of displays of extreme fear, yelling, and arm waving while asleep. Some incidents of sleepwalking frequently accompany these behaviors. It is also important to differentiate sleep terrors from nightmares. Usually, people who have a nightmare wake up and can remember at least some details of their bad dream. In contrast, those who suffer a sleep terror episode stay asleep, and when they later awaken they are not likely to remember anything about the incident.

Besides being afraid and shouting, other symptoms of sleep terrors may include kicking at the bed or other furniture, running from room to room as if being chased, striking out at people or pets, sweating profusely, breathing heavily, having a racing pulse, and being hard to awaken. Indeed, "you can't shake a person out of sleep terror," Foldvary-Schaefer cautions, "and the frightened sleeper will not respond to your voice no matter how loudly you speak. The best thing to do is to stand nearby and make sure the person is not injured during the episode. Of course, this might not be possible if the person is thrashing or violent, which is more common in adults. Attempts to restrain the sleeper may provoke more aggressive responses."[50]

Treatment for sleep terrors varies from doctor to doctor and depends on the severity of the problem. Mild cases, which outnumber the severe ones, may need no major intervention at all, as explained by the sleep specialists at the Mayo Clinic (with its main offices in Rochester, Minnesota):

> Treatment for sleep terrors isn't usually necessary. If your child has a sleep terror, simply wait it out. You might gently restrain your child and try to get him or her back into bed. Speak softly and calmly. Shaking your child or shouting may make things worse. If the sleep terrors are associated with an underlying medical or mental health condition or another sleep disorder, treatment is aimed at the underlying problem. If stress or anxiety seems to be contributing to the sleep terrors, your doctor may suggest meeting with a therapist or counselor. Cognitive behavior therapy, hypnosis, biofeedback, and relaxation therapy may help. Medication is rarely used to treat sleep terrors, particularly for children.[51]

Fight or Flight in the Night

Similar in some ways to sleep terrors, but more extreme and potentially dangerous, is REM sleep behavior disorder,

In a Panic Each Night

A young boy named Caleb woke up most nights in a state of fear. His mother, Sandy, took him to his pediatrician, who soon recommended a sleep specialist. A doctor at a noted sleep clinic determined that the boy suffered from the sleep disorder called sleep terrors. Part of Caleb's case history follows.

> [His] blood-curdling scream jarred his mother from a deep sleep. She ran down the hall, threw open the door to her 7-year-old son's bedroom, and found him sitting upright in his bed—eyes wide open, breathing like he'd been playing tag, rocking back and forth, and mumbling incoherently. "Caleb, wake up! It's okay—I'm here." Caleb looked through his mother as though she were a ghost. The eerie disconnect worried Sandy. She had been certain that after tucking him into bed more than an hour ago, he would sleep through the night this time. . . . Caleb's episodes are happening more frequently. The previous week he woke up almost every night—always about an hour after going to bed. The episodes worry Sandy because Caleb never remembers the horrible incidents that scare him into a panic each night.

Quoted in Nancy Foldvary-Schaefer. *The Cleveland Clinic Guide to Sleep Disorders.* New York: Kaplan, 2009, pp. 131–132.

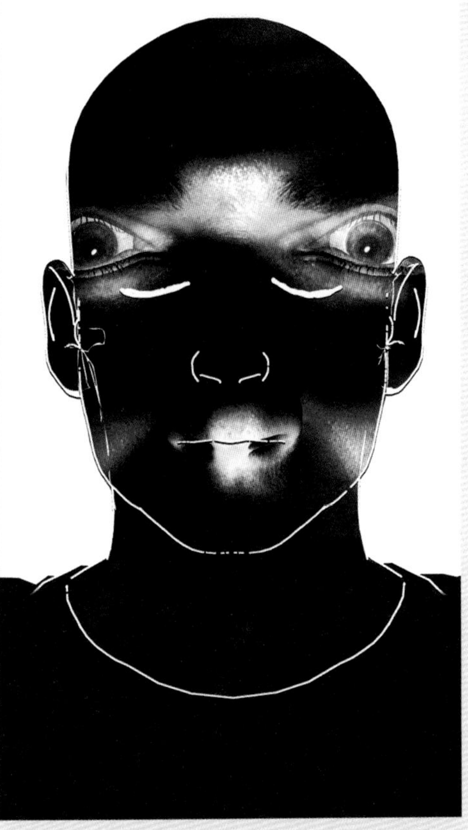

Sleep terrors are most common among children three to twelve years of age. The disorder tends to disappear during adolescence.

frequently referred to by its initials, RBD. The most colorful brief description of this exceptionally bizarre problem is by Schenck, who writes:

> What if you find out that you become transformed in your sleep from a peaceful person to an attacking monster? A bit like in werewolf mythology, people with REM sleep behavior disorder, or RBD, seem to become wholly different creatures in their sleep. [For] those with RBD . . . the rules of sleep don't apply—with frightening consequences. Those afflicted with RBD lack the protective mechanism [that] immobilizes them during REM slecp. Therefore, their bodies are free to get up and act out their dreams. The scenario is made worse because RBD dream-enactment does not involve one's average dreams—[instead] they're pointedly more vivid, intense, physically active, confrontational, aggressive, and violent, with classic fight-or-flight scenarios.[52]

The most common treatment for RBD is the drug clonazepam, which eliminates symptoms in about 90 percent of cases.

Thus, those with RBD—who are more often men than women—have a serious and scary problem. In their sleep

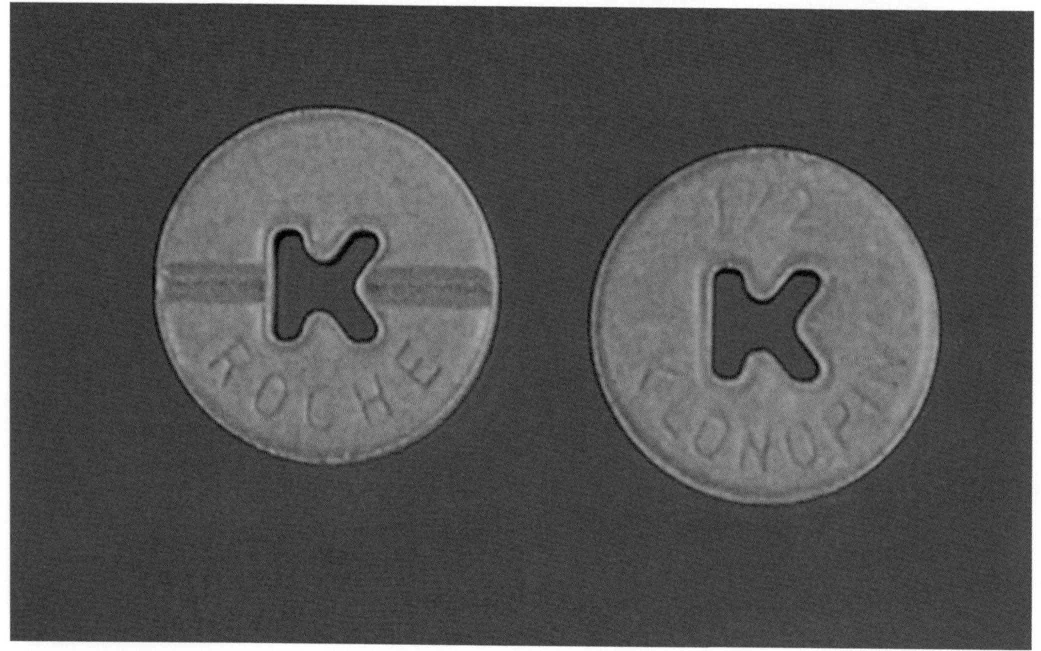

they are driven to attack and even to try to kill wild animals or human intruders. Unfortunately for all involved, those beasts and attackers are in reality most often their bed partners, who suddenly find themselves on the receiving end of verbal abuse and/or dangerous physical assault. One documented case was that of a World War II veteran who dreamed about fighting off attacking enemy soldiers. While sleeping, he violently kicked his bedpost, mistaking it for one of those attackers. Another RBD sleeper thought a hideous monster was chasing him. Desperately trying to get away, he punched his wife in her rib cage, not realizing, of course, whom he was striking. In a similar incident, another man with RBD choked his wife (who fortunately managed to break loose), thinking he was fighting a wild animal. Still another man with RBD dreamed he was one of King Arthur's knights dashing through a castle and manifested it by running madly around his house while asleep.

In order to diagnose RBD with certainty, sleep specialists usually call for a formal sleep study to be performed in a sleep center, where the person can be observed closely while he or she sleeps. This is because RBD can easily be confused with other parasomnias, including sleep terrors. If the diagnosis confirms that the culprit is RBD, the most common treatment is to prescribe a medicine such as clonazepam. That drug decreases or even eliminates the symptoms of this violent disorder in about 90 percent of cases. Experts also recommend doing whatever is necessary to make the person's bedroom and nearby rooms as safe as possible by taking away all breakable and sharp objects.

In fact, this same advice can be applied to several other parasomnias, including sleepwalking and sleep terrors. Until a person who regularly wrestles with them is treated by a medical professional, safety is the best practice.

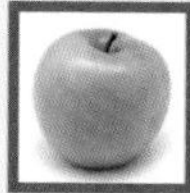

CHAPTER 5

Finding Paths to Better Sleep

Sleep disorders are not only uncomfortable, unhealthful, and in some cases dangerous, they are also signs that the individual is not able to achieve normal, healthy sleep patterns. Every person with such a problem would like to find one or more paths to better sleep. One of those paths is adopting good sleep hygiene, a collection of practices and habits that promote regular, normal sleep. Depending on the type and severity of one's sleep problem, seeking help from a doctor might be an important step, too. Among the possible therapies a physician might prescribe are various kinds of sleeping pills and other drugs, and the patient needs to think about the possible side effects that accompany that approach. Still another possible path a person with a sleep disorder might end up taking is undergoing a sleep study in a sleep center.

These and similar approaches to healthful sleep are sometimes referred to as sleep strategies. Because individual personalities, backgrounds, settings, and sleep problems vary, one person's sleep strategy may not work well for many others. So finding just the right combination of therapies is often a matter of trial and error. "Good sleep strategies are essential to deep, restorative sleep you can count on, night after night," the sleep researchers at Helpguide say. "By learning to avoid common enemies of sleep and trying out a variety of healthy sleep-promoting techniques, you can discover your personal prescription to a good night's rest. The key is to experiment. What works for some might not work as well for others. It's important to find the sleep strategies that work best for you."[53]

Good Sleep Hygiene

All doctors, sleep specialists, and sleep clinics agree that one of the basic strategies a person with a sleep problem should adopt is practicing good sleep hygiene. In fact, the first thing most doctors do when interviewing a new sleep-disordered patient is ask about his or her sleeping habits. Adopting proper sleep hygiene may not by itself solve or cure a person's sleep problem or problems. But medical authorities see it as a useful baseline, or starting point, in any attempt to help someone learn to sleep better.

Good sleep habits are important in fighting sleep disorders. Regularity—that is, retiring and rising at the same times each day, including weekends—is especially important.

First and foremost on the list of good sleep habits is trying to go to bed at the same time each night, even on weekends. One should also attempt to get up at roughly the same

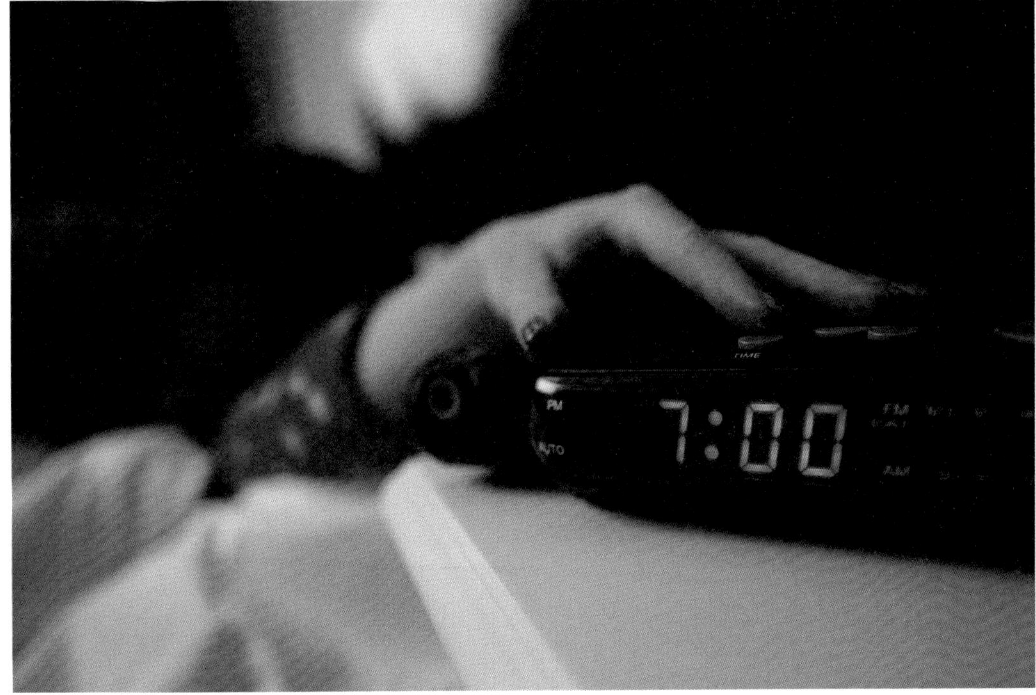

time each morning, including on weekends when possible. Sleep experts say that adopting this regimen helps the body maintain a strong, healthy sleep-wake rhythm. They also say that a person should aim at getting at least seven and a half hours of sleep a night, and a little more if possible. (Some people need as much as nine hours of sleep a night.) Moreover, they should try not to take naps during the day, at least on a regular basis. This is because taking naps habitually can cause someone to sleep less at night and thereby throw off his or her healthy sleep-wake rhythm.

People should also try to sleep in a room that is dark, quiet, and as relaxing as possible. One way to make the room darker is to get window blinds or shades that are opaque and keep most light out. Also, the temperature should be comfortable—that is, not too hot or too cold—for the individual sleeper. Some people find it easier and more restful to sleep in a warm room, whereas others prefer a cooler temperature. People who like it cooler sometimes open a window a little, even in the winter, in order to keep the temperature where they like it.

Experts also recommend stopping activities such as exercising, watching television, and listening to music a little while before bedtime. This allows both the body and the mind to relax prior to the onset of sleep. Evidence shows it is best to stop exercising at least three to four hours before bedtime. Otherwise, the body may feel overstimulated, which can make it harder to get to sleep.

Some Helpful Hygiene Tips

One should also avoid eating a big meal shortly before bedtime, sleep specialists say, because this forces the digestive tract into overdrive. While the stomach and intestines are working hard to digest food, a person will find it harder both to fall and stay asleep. It is also a good idea to avoid alcohol in the evening because it has been shown to diminish sleep quality. Similarly, caffeine—from coffee, tea, chocolate bars, and other drinks and foods—and nicotine—from smoking or chewing tobacco—should be avoided before bedtime. The reason is that these substances are stimulants, which can interfere with falling asleep.

A Snack Before Bedtime

Although sleep experts say that a person should not eat a big meal shortly before bedtime, they point out that having a small snack can actually be beneficial. Melinda Smith and the other sleep researchers at Helpguide explain:

> For some people, a light snack before bed can help promote sleep. When you pair tryptophan-containing foods with carbohydrates, it may help calm the brain and allow you to sleep better. For others, eating before bed can lead to indigestion and make sleeping more difficult. Experiment with your food habits to determine your optimum evening meals and snacks. If you need a bedtime snack, try: half a turkey sandwich, a small bowl of whole-grain, low-sugar cereal, granola with low-fat milk or yogurt, or a banana.

Melinda Smith, Lawrence Robinson, and Robert Segal. "How to Sleep Better." Helpguide. www.helpguide.org/life/sleep_tips.htm.

Research shows that eating a small snack before bedtime can help one to sleep.

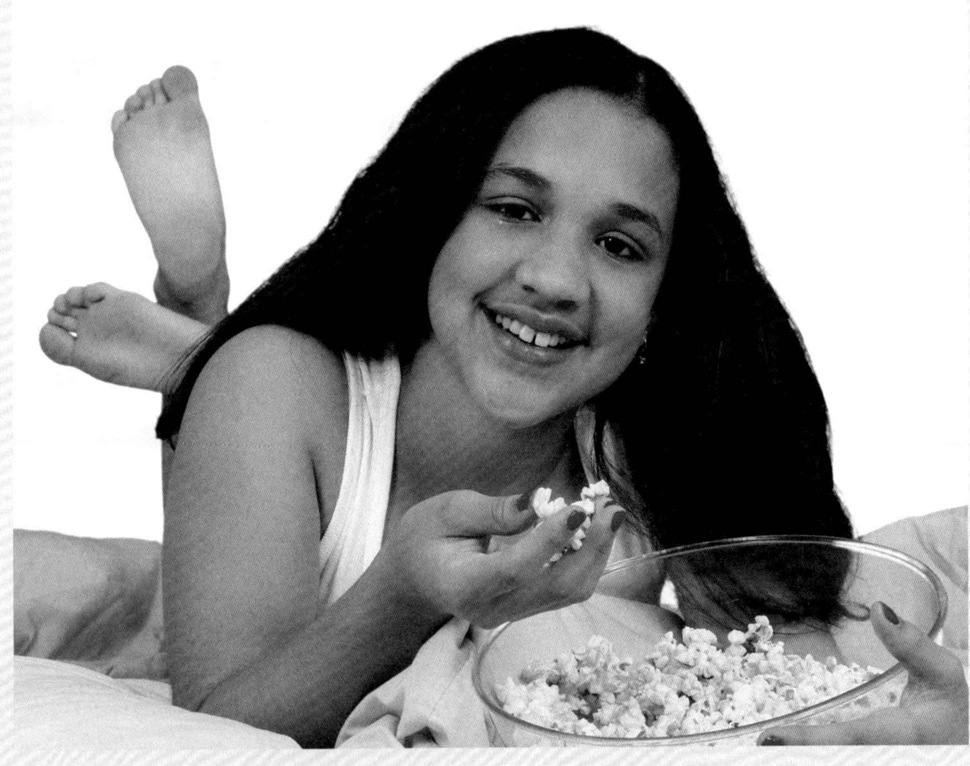

Louis R. Chanin offers some other helpful tips on achieving and maintaining good sleep hygiene. "If light is a problem," he writes, "try a sleeping mask. If noise is a problem, try earplugs, a fan, or a 'white noise' machine to cover up the sounds." Also, he says, "Avoid using your bed for anything other than sleep or sex. If you can't fall asleep and don't feel drowsy, get up and read or do something that is not overly stimulating until you feel sleepy. If you find yourself lying awake worrying about things, try making a to-do list before you go to bed. This may help you to not focus on those worries overnight."[54]

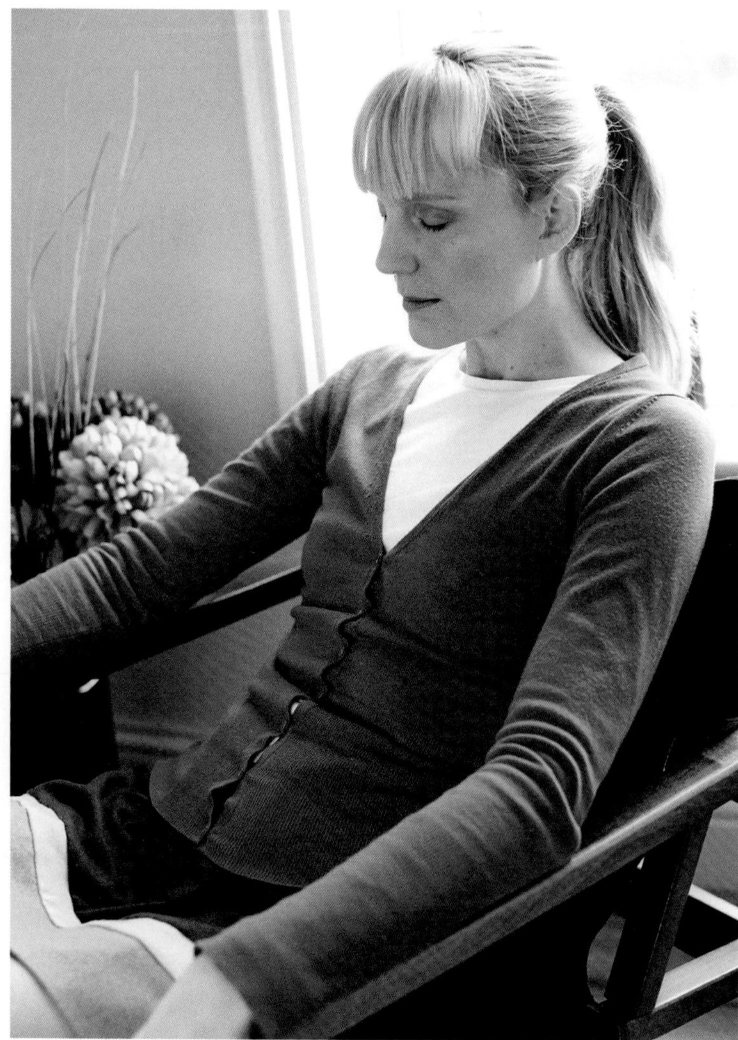

Finding healthy ways to manage stress can help insomnia sufferers restore normal sleep patterns.

Finally, people can improve their sleep habits by learning to manage stress better. Numerous medical studies have shown that stress, in one form or another, is common and widespread in modern society and that nearly everyone is faced with stressful situations from time to time. Without a doubt, the more stress one is forced to deal with, the harder it is for him or her to get regular, restful sleep. The doctors at the Mayo Clinic offer the following advice on getting a good start on stress management:

> When you have too much to do—and too much to think about—your sleep is likely to suffer. To help restore peace to your life, consider healthy ways to manage stress. Start with the basics, such as getting organized, setting priorities and delegating tasks. Give yourself permission to take a break when you need one. Share a good laugh with an old friend. Before bed, jot down what's on your mind and then set it aside for tomorrow.[55]

HEALTH FACT

According to the NIH, the notion that someone's body can easily and quickly adjust to different sleep schedules is a myth.

Keeping a Sleep Diary

A doctor or other specialist who recommends maintaining such healthy sleep habits may suggest that a patient keep a sleep diary for a couple of weeks or perhaps longer. Sometimes a person who is concerned about his or her sleep habits may try keeping a sleep diary on his or her own initiative. Either way, this can be very helpful because it forces the person to take a close, detailed look at his or her daily sleep-related activities. Often, people do not remember exactly what they did the day or week or month before. So seeing it in writing can provide a helpful reminder, reveal insight into one's own habits, and to some degree put one's life in a new and refreshing perspective.

A number of medical and health organizations that specialize in sleep-related topics offer sample templates of sleep diaries. Like most, the one offered by the National Sleep

Foundation is a chart divided into rows of squares for entering data. It lists general activities, such as "I went to bed last night at," "I got out of bed this morning at," and "Last night I slept a total of" across the top. The individual days—"Day 1," "Day 2,"[56] and so forth—are arranged vertically on the left side. By checking the diary after, say, two weeks, a person can see that on Day 3 he or she went to bed at 11:00 P.M., for example; that on Day 9 he or she woke up at 5:30 A.M.; and that on Day 12 he or she got a total of seven hours of sleep. There are also rows of squares to show whether and when the person drank alcohol or caffeinated beverages, exercised, or took prescribed medicine.

After a while, people's sleep diaries will show, almost at a glance, whether they are practicing healthy sleep habits. Patterns will emerge that indicate the areas in which individuals are doing well, as well as the areas in which they need improvement. Regarding the latter, they may need to cut down on caffeinated drinks before bed. Or they might need to increase the number of hours they sleep on the weekends. Another benefit of keeping a sleep diary is that people can compare their ongoing habits with how good or bad they feel on certain days. If they do feel tired or listless one day, the reasons for it will likely be evident in the diary entries for the night before.

Pills and Other Sleep Medicines

Some people not only keep sleep diaries on their own, they also take pills and other medicines bought over the counter in hopes of curing insomnia or some other problem that interferes with proper sleep. Sleep experts say this is usually not a good idea, for several reasons. First, because such a drug has not been prescribed by a doctor, it may not be the best medicine for the job, or it may not work at all. Second, whether it is obtained over the counter or prescribed by a doctor, no drug can *cure* insomnia or another sleep disorder. At best, it can lessen the severity of one or more symptoms.

Third, and especially important, individuals may already be taking medicines for other reasons, and some of these medicines may counteract the effects of the ones they take to help them sleep. Indeed, many over-the-counter drugs that people take for a host of different medical problems actually make it more difficult for someone to fall asleep. According to the NIH:

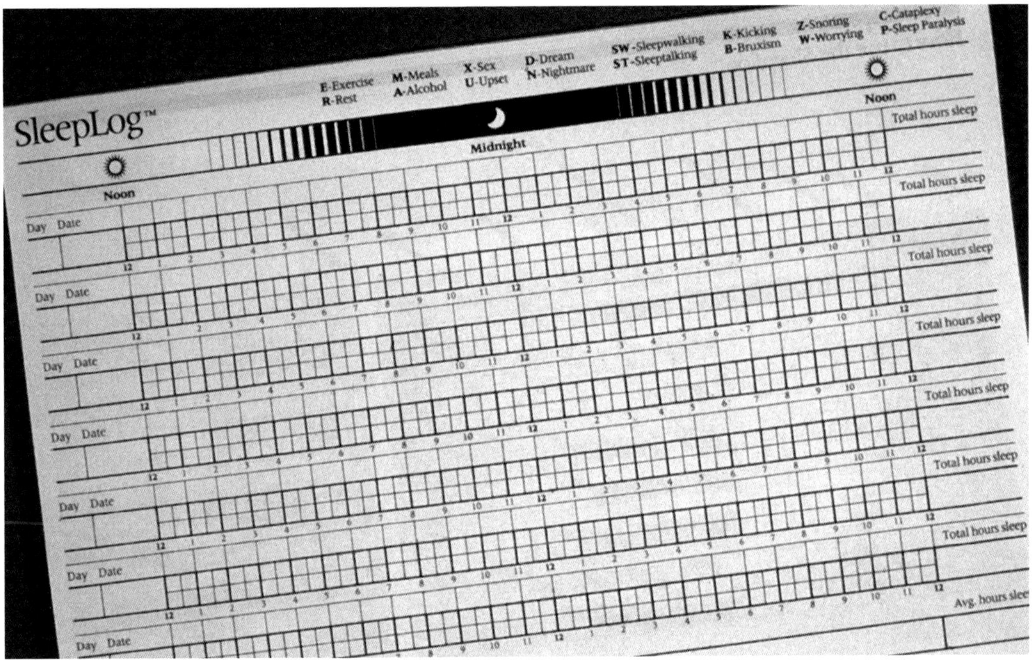

> Certain commonly used prescription and over-the-counter medicines contain ingredients that can keep you awake. These ingredients include decongestants and steroids. Many medicines taken to relieve headaches contain caffeine. Heart and blood pressure medications known as beta blockers can make it difficult to fall asleep and cause more awakenings during the night. People who have chronic asthma or bronchitis also have more problems falling asleep and staying asleep than healthy people, either because of their breathing difficulties or because of the medicines they take. Other chronic painful or uncomfortable conditions—such as arthritis, congestive heart failure, and sickle cell anemia—can disrupt sleep, too.[57]

It is much more effective and healthy, therefore, to make sure that any pills and other medicines one takes to aid proper sleep be prescribed by a doctor. The National Sleep

Sleep researchers use sleep logs and patients' sleep diaries to help sleep-disordered clients to take a closer look at their sleep-related activities and habits.

Foundation and other reputable sleep authorities say that when taken as instructed, certain drugs prescribed by physicians as sleep aids *can* safely treat insomnia and some other conditions. Still, the patient must understand that those medicines cannot cure such conditions. Also, in order to be even minimally effective, they need to be taken exactly as instructed. If not used correctly, they can actually make the condition worse, or they might even create unexpected and unwanted problems.

There is also the potential of becoming dependent on a sleep aid, whether it is bought over the counter or prescribed by a doctor. Certainly, anyone who has a history of addiction to alcohol, cocaine, or some other drug faces an increased risk of becoming dependent on a sleep medicine. For that reason, it is imperative to tell the doctor about any prior or existing addiction problems one might have. Finally, no sleep aid should be consumed along with alcohol, particularly before driving or operating machinery. Mixing alcohol with certain drugs can cause a dangerous or even life-threatening reaction.

Alternative Therapies

In addition to traditional drugs and other medicines prescribed by doctors, various herbal and dietary supplements and alternative remedies have been used by people with insomnia or other sleep disorders. Most are advertised as "natural," which to many people suggests they are healthy and safe to consume. But while this is likely true of some of them, a number of others may have side effects that range from mild to severe, depending on how much of the substance the person takes. One common side effect of such alternative medicines is significant interference with, or canceling out the effects of, vitamins and/or other drugs the person may already be taking. Thus, to be safe it is a good idea to check with a doctor or pharmacist first before beginning a regimen of alternative remedies.

At least a few of those remedies do show promise in treating insomnia and perhaps a few other sleep disorders. Of these, the best known is melatonin. Melatonin is a hormone marketed over the counter as an aid to treat the symptoms of insomnia. The human body produces small amounts of melatonin naturally, mostly in the hours just after sundown and in smaller amounts from midnight until dawn. The problem is that some people may produce smaller amounts of the hormone than other people do, which might negatively affect sleep. Tests indicate that taking melatonin supplements does help some insomniacs sleep better. However, to date, no solid evidence has been found to show that these supplements work for everyone. Moreover, as sleep specialists at the Mayo Clinic point out, "the long-term safety of melatonin is unknown."[58]

Another widely marketed alternative sleep aid is an herb called valerian. Because it has mild sedative properties, it has helped some people who have trouble getting to sleep. However, it has not yet been well studied, the Mayo Clinic cautions. "In addition," the Mayo Clinic staff adds, it "has been associated with liver damage in some people, though it's not clear if valerian was the cause of the damage."[59]

Acupuncture has been found to be moderately successful in treating sleep disorders while having no bad side effects.

Another alternative treatment for insomnia has proved to be at least moderately effective without having any significant negative side effects. It is the ancient Chinese medical treatment of acupuncture. In a typical session, a medical practitioner trained in the procedure inserts a number of

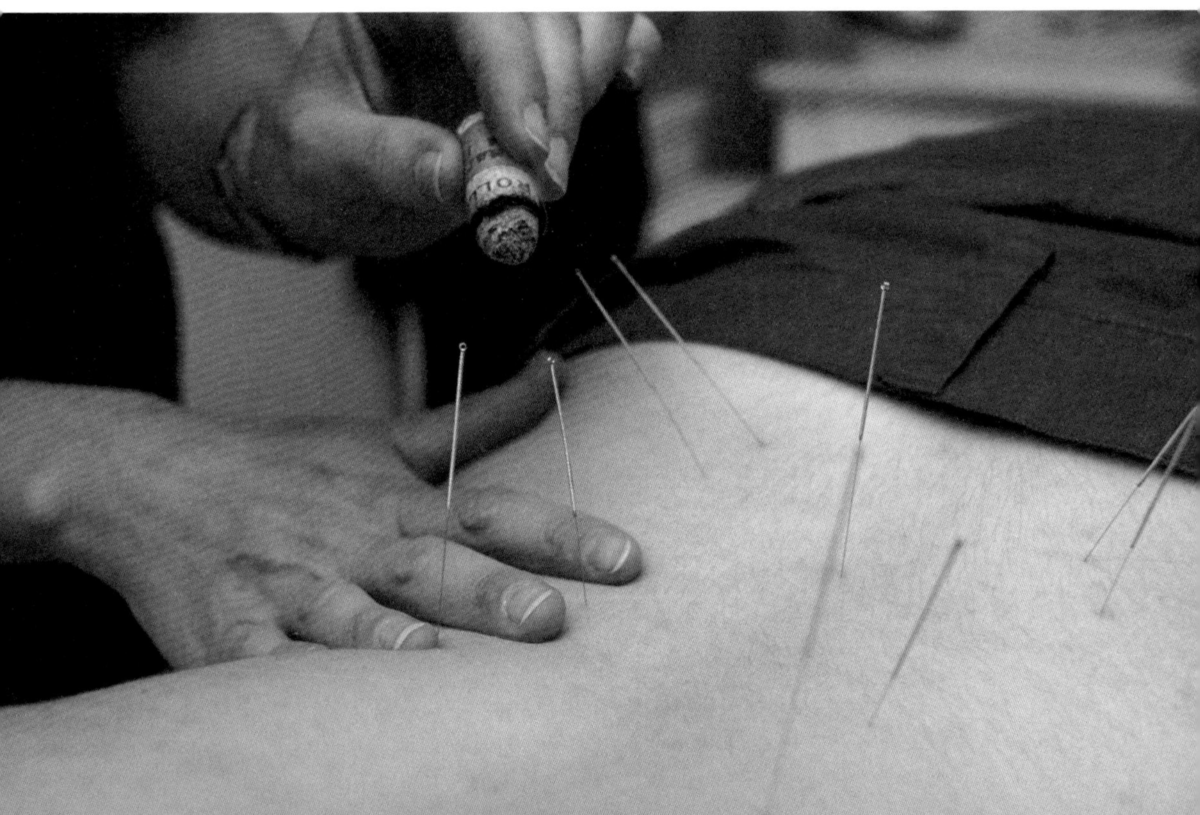

Taking Part in Research

Research into sleep and sleep disorders is ongoing. Such research requires that clinical trials and studies be done, and test subjects are always needed. The NIH provides the following information for people interested in participating:

> If you participate in clinical research, the research will be explained to you in detail, you will be given a chance to ask questions, and you will be asked to provide written permission. You may not directly benefit from the results of the clinical research you participate in, but the information gathered will help others and will add to scientific knowledge. . . . If you're thinking about participating in a clinical study, you may have questions about the purpose of the study, the types of tests and treatment involved, how participation will affect your daily life, and whether any costs are involved. Your doctor may be able to answer some of your questions and help you find clinical studies in which you can participate. You also can visit the following websites to learn about being in a study and to search for clinical trials being done on your disorder:
>
> www.clinicaltrials.gov, http://clinicalresearch.nih.gov,
>
> www.nhlbi.nih.gov/studies/index.htm.

National Institutes of Health. *Your Guide to Healthy Sleep.* Washington, DC: National Institutes of Health, 2011, p. 59.

extremely thin needles in the patient's skin at specific spots on the body. For reasons that are not well understood, acupuncture treatment has been successful in providing relief for some medical conditions, including insomnia. According to the National Center for Biotechnology Information in Washington, D.C., "Clinical studies have shown that acupuncture may have a beneficial effect on insomnia" comparable to that of some "Western medications."[60]

Roles of Doctors and Sleep Clinics

Over the years, many people with sleep disorders who tried alternative medicines or other over-the-counter products found no relief using them. Others suffered from symptoms of such problems for years, never tried any sort of treatment, and eventually became sleep deprived and miserable. According to leading sleep experts, the best course for individuals in both of these groups is to see a doctor, either in his or her office setting or in a hospital. Depending on the nature or severity of the case, the doctor may then recommend other options.

The CDC, NHLBI, National Sleep Foundation, Mayo Clinic, and other organizations that deal with sleep problems have listed the general situations in which a person should seek professional help for those problems. First, they say, if someone with insomnia or another sleep disorder has tried to treat it with nonprescription, over-the-counter medicines that did not help, he or she should go to a doctor. The same is true of a person whose sleep problem is causing significant difficulties or crises at work or school. Certainly, it is time to go to a physician or hospital if one experiences symptoms such as shortness of breath, constant headaches, or frequent chest pains. Finally, if a sleep problem affects someone nearly every night and he or she never gets any better, seeing a doctor is a must. In the words of medical writer Michelle Andrews:

> If you have sleeping difficulties for more than a month, consider seeing a doctor, preferably at a clinic that specializes in sleep disorders. (To find one in your area, you can go to sleepcenters.org.) A specialist may do a complete work-up and identify medical problems that have been keeping you from getting the restful shut-eye you need. If you turn out to have sleep apnea, a doctor may fit you with a device that delivers pressurized air through the nose and helps keep your airway open. For other problems, a sleep specialist may work with you to change behaviors that can perpetuate insomnia. The practitioner may urge you to get out

of bed whenever you're unable to sleep, for example, or may temporarily limit the number of hours you spend in bed to help you develop more consolidated, stable sleep patterns. He or she may prescribe sleeping pills as well.[61]

Doing a Sleep Study

In addition, if it seems warranted, the medical professional may urge the person to undergo a sleep study at a sleep center or clinic. According to the National Sleep Foundation, when getting ready for a sleep study, the patient should make sure he or she knows what to do, or what not to do, beforehand. Typical questions the person might want to ask a member of the center's staff include:

> Does it matter if I take a nap the day before or the day of the study? Should I refrain from drinking coffee, tea, or other caffeinated products, or energy drinks? If so, for how many hours before my test? What can I eat before the study? In addition to caffeinated products, are there any other foods/beverages that I should avoid? Should I avoid stimulants, alcohol, or sedatives? What about other prescription and non-prescription medications, and/or dietary or herbal supplements?[62]

HEALTH FACT

The theory behind acupuncture states that the body's functions are governed by an invisible energy known as chi and that the needles correct imbalances that arise. Scientists have so far been unable to verify the existence of chi, though the procedure seems to work in some cases.

The person might also want to ask what he or she should bring to wear during the sleep study and whether it will be all right for a family member to remain with him or her during the test. Another common concern is whether the person will be allowed to take a shower and dress for work on the morning following the test. A number of these situations and rules may differ from one sleep clinic to another.

In the study itself, the patient will go to bed in a room at the clinic at about the same time he or she does

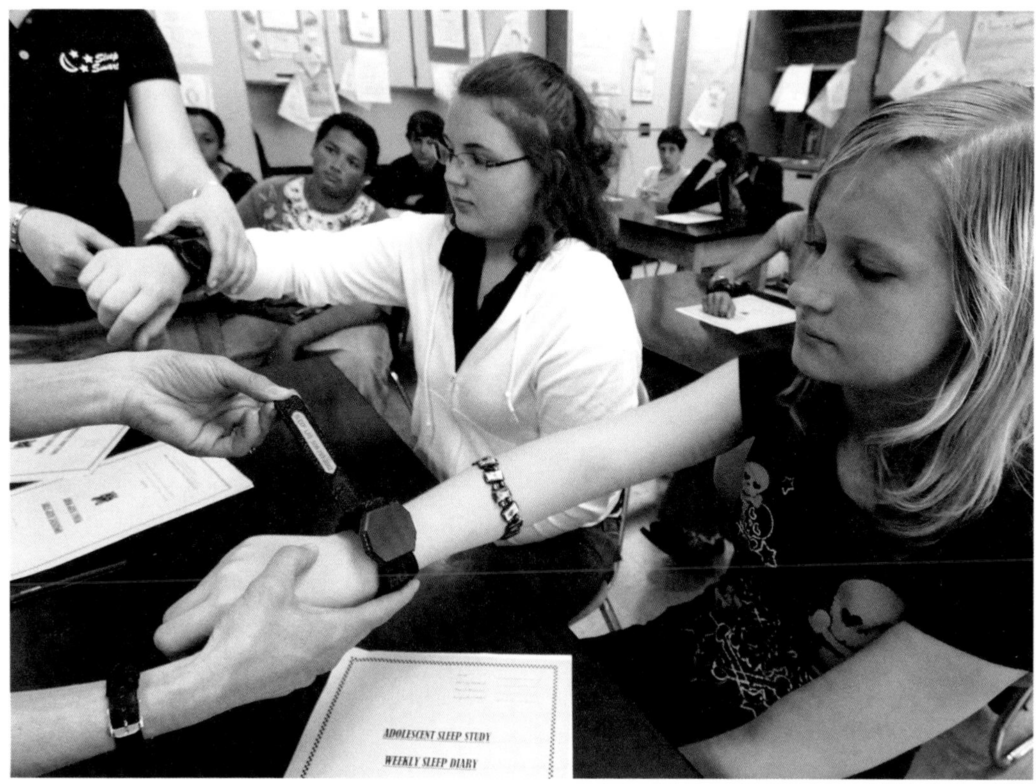

Teens participating in a sleep study are fitted with activgraphs, devices that will monitor their movements during sleep.

most nights. Just before nodding off, a technician will attach electrodes and monitors to the person's legs, chest, and head. (This does not hurt.) While the person sleeps, the technician will record his or her heart rhythm and breathing, brain wave activity, eye movements, and other important bodily functions. The next morning, the data from these recordings will be given to a sleep doctor. The doctor will evaluate the data and shortly afterward formulate a diagnosis and suggest a potential treatment. From that point on, the sleep doctor may continue to see the patient until the problem is resolved to the satisfaction of both. That physician will send information about the sleep study results, diagnosis, and treatment to the patient's regular doctor to keep him or her in the loop.

Even if a person with sleep problems does not end up needing to undergo a sleep study, seeing his or her doctor remains a crucial and highly recommended step. As Lawrence J. Epstein strongly emphasizes, trying to treat such problems on one's own is rarely successful and might in some cases be a health risk. "If you have trouble sleeping," he says, "I encourage you to seek help. It's important not to give up and remember that help is available. Whatever the cause of your sleep difficulty . . . I can't tell you how many times patients who have struggled for years ultimately experience major improvement when their problem is correctly diagnosed and treated. Better sleep means better health. Sleep well."[63]

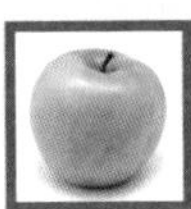

NOTES

Introduction: Dispelling a Famous Sleep Myth

1. Quoted in Piotr A. Wozniak. "Polyphasic Sleep: Facts and Myths." Super Memory. www.supermemo.com/articles/polyphasic.htm.
2. Quoted in Brett McKay and Kate McKay. "The Napping Habits of 8 Famous Men." Art of Manliness, March 14, 2011. http://artofmanliness.com/2011/03/14/the-napping-habits-of-8-famous-men.
3. Quoted in McKay and McKay. "The Napping Habits of 8 Famous Men."
4. Wozniak. "Polyphasic Sleep."
5. Carlos H. Schenck. *Sleep*. New York: Avery, 2008, p. xvi.

Chapter 1: Why Sleep Is Vital to Everyone

6. Schenck. *Sleep*, p. 1.
7. *Merriam-Webster*. "Sleep." www.merriam-webster.com/medical/sleep.
8. Melinda Smith, Lawrence Robinson, and Robert Segal. "How Much Sleep Do You Need?" Helpguide. www.helpguide.org/life/sleeping.htm.
9. Stuart F. Quan, ed. "The Characteristics of Sleep." Healthy Sleep, December 18, 2007. http://healthysleep.med.harvard.edu/healthy/science/what/characteristics.
10. National Heart, Lung, and Blood Institute. "Why Is Sleep Important?" www.nhlbi.nih.gov/health/health-topics/topics/sdd/why.html.
11. Centers for Disease Control and Prevention. "Sleep and Sleep Disorders." www.cdc.gov/sleep.
12. Schenck. *Sleep*, p. 4.
13. Elizabeth Weise. "Gene Found That Lets People Get By on 6 Hours of Sleep." ABCNews.com. http://abcnews.go.com/Technology/story?id=8322077&page=1#.UOHal3ez7ak.
14. Weise. "Gene Found That Lets People Get By on 6 Hours of Sleep."
15. Smith et al. "How Much Sleep Do You Need?"
16. William Dement. "Sleepless at Stanford." Sleep Well. www.stanford.edu/~dement/sleepless.html.

Chapter 2: The Chief Sleep Disorder: Insomnia

17. Michelle Andrews. "Can't Sleep? Why Insomnia Shouldn't Be Ignored." *U.S. News & World Report*, March 2, 2009. http://health.usnews.com/health-news/family-health/sleep/articles/2009/03/02/cant-sleep-why-insomnia-shouldnt-be-ignored.
18. Max Hirshkowitz and Patricia B. Smith. *Sleep Disorders for Dummies*. Indianapolis, IN: Wiley, 2004, p. 62.
19. National Heart, Lung, and Blood Institute. "Who Is at Risk for Insomnia?" www.nhlbi.nih.gov/health/health-topics/topics/inso/atrisk.html.
20. Hirshkowitz and Smith. *Sleep Disorders for Dummies*, p. 67.
21. Nancy Foldvary-Schaefer. *The Cleveland Clinic Guide to Sleep Disorders*. New York: Kaplan, 2009, p. 112.
22. Phyllis C. Zee. "Insomnia and Falls in the Elderly." Medscape. www.medscape.org/viewarticle/518832.
23. Herbert Ross, Keri Brenner, and Burton Goldberg. *Sleep Disorders*. Tiburon, CA: AlternativeMedicine.com, 2000, p. 51.
24. William Dement and Christopher Vaughan. *The Promise of Sleep*. New York: Dell, 1999, pp. 136–137.
25. Dement and Vaughan. *The Promise of Sleep*, p. 137.
26. Foldvary-Schaefer. *The Cleveland Clinic Guide to Sleep Disorders*, p. 113.
27. Theresa F. DiGeronimo. *Insomnia: 50 Essential Things to Do*. New York: Plume, 1997, pp. 32–33.
28. National Heart, Lung, and Blood Institute. "How to Discuss Sleep with Your Doctor." www.nhlbi.nih.gov/health/health-topics/topics/sdd/howto.html.
29. Louis R. Chanin. "An Overview of Insomnia." WebMD, July 29, 2012. www.webmd.com/sleep-disorders/guide/insomnia-symptoms-and-causes.
30. Andrews. "Can't Sleep? Why Insomnia Shouldn't Be Ignored."

Chapter 3: Other Common Sleep Disorders

31. Foldvary-Schaefer. *The Cleveland Clinic Guide to Sleep Disorders*, p. 50.
32. Dement and Vaughan. *The Promise of Sleep*, p. 168.
33. Schenck. *Sleep*, p. 37.
34. National Heart, Lung, and Blood Institute. "What Is Sleep Apnea?" www.nhlbi.nih.gov/health/health-topics/topics/sleepapnea.
35. Dement and Vaughan. *The Promise of Sleep*, p. 172.
36. Dement and Vaughan. *The Promise of Sleep*, p. 172.
37. Hirshkowitz and Smith. *Sleep Disorders for Dummies*, p. 89.
38. RLS Foundation. "About RLS: Is There a Known Cause of RLS?"

www.rls.org/page.aspx?pid=543 #13.
39. Lawrence J. Epstein. *The Harvard Medical School Guide to a Good Night's Sleep.* New York: McGraw-Hill, 2007, p. 153.
40. Melinda Smith, Lawrence Robinson, and Robert Segal. "Sleep Disorders and Sleeping Problems." Helpguide. www.helpguide.org /life/sleep_disorders.htm.
41. National Sleep Foundation. "Narcolepsy and Sleep." www.sleepfoundation.org/article/sleep-related -problems/narcolepsy-and-sleep.
42. Epstein. *The Harvard Medical School Guide to a Good Night's Sleep*, pp. 156–157.
43. Epstein. *The Harvard Medical School Guide to a Good Night's Sleep*, p. 157.
44. Interview with the author, January 4, 2013.

Chapter 4: Weird Behaviors While Sleeping

45. Hirshkowitz and Smith. *Sleep Disorders for Dummies*, pp. 231–232.
46. Quoted in Schenck. *Sleep*, p. 114.
47. Schenck. *Sleep*, pp. 116–117.
48. Ross et al. *Sleep Disorders*, p. 46.
49. Foldvary-Schaefer. *The Cleveland Clinic Guide to Sleep Disorders*, p. 134.
50. Foldvary-Schaefer. *The Cleveland Clinic Guide to Sleep Disorders*, p. 135.
51. Mayo Clinic staff. "Sleep Terrors: Treatments and Drugs." Mayo Clinic. www.mayoclinic.com/ health/night-terrors/DS01016/ DSECTION=treatments-and -drugs.
52. Schenck. *Sleep*, pp. 197–198.

Chapter 5: Finding Paths to Better Sleep

53. Melinda Smith, Lawrence Robinson, and Robert Segal. "How to Sleep Better." Helpguide. www.helpguide.org/life/sleep_tips.htm.
54. Louis R. Chanin. "An Overview of Insomnia: Good Sleep Habits for Beating Insomnia." www.webmd .com/sleep-disorders/guide/insomnia-symptoms-and-causes?page =2.
55. Mayo Clinic staff. "Sleep Tips: Seven Steps to Better Sleep." Mayo Clinic. www.mayoclinic.com /health/sleep/HQ01387/NSECTIONGROUP=2.
56. National Sleep Foundation. "National Sleep Foundation Sleep Diary." http://sleep.buffalo.edu /sleepdiary.pdf.
57. National Institutes of Health. *Your Guide to Healthy Sleep.* Washington, DC: National Institutes of Health, 2011, pp. 25–26.
58. Mayo Clinic staff. "Alternative Medicine." Mayo Clinic. www .mayoclinic.com/health/insomnia /DS00187/DSECTION=alternative -medicine.
59. Mayo Clinic staff. "Alternative Medicine."

60. National Center for Biotechnology Information. "Acupuncture for Treatment of Insomnia: A Systematic Review of Randomized Controlled Trials." www.ncbi.nlm.nih.gov/pubmed/19922248.
61. Andrews. "Can't Sleep? Why Insomnia Shouldn't Be Ignored."
62. National Sleep Foundation, "Sleep Studies." http://www.sleepfoundation.org/article/sleep-topics/sleep-studies
63. Epstein. *The Harvard Medical School Guide to a Good Night's Sleep*, p. 257.

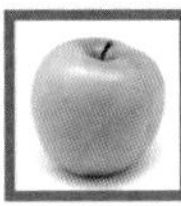

GLOSSARY

bruxism: Teeth grinding; a sleep disorder in which a person repeatedly clenches the teeth while sleeping.

cataplexy: A loss of muscle control, often associated with the sleep disorder narcolepsy.

chronic: Persistent or long-lasting.

continuous positive airway pressure device (CPAP): A mask that helps those with sleep apnea keep their throats open.

depression (especially clinical or chronic depression): Prolonged, deep sadness.

insomnia: The most common sleep disorder, characterized by difficulty falling or staying asleep.

narcolepsy: A sleep disorder in which a person suddenly falls asleep during the daytime.

nocturnal enuresis: Bed-wetting; a sleep disorder in which a person urinates while asleep.

non-REM sleep: Consisting of four stages, the sleep state that precedes REM sleep.

REM: Rapid eye movement; a physical trait of the fifth sleep stage, REM sleep

REM sleep behavior disorder (RBD): A sleep disorder in which a person performs violent acts while sleeping.

restless legs syndrome (RLS): A sleep disorder characterized by odd and uncomfortable sensations in the legs.

sleep apnea: A sleep disorder in which a person repeatedly stops breathing while asleep.

sleep debt: The amount of sleep the body is owed when a person gets too little sleep in a given sleep session.

sleep terrors (or night terrors): A sleep disorder in which a person exhibits extreme fear while asleep.

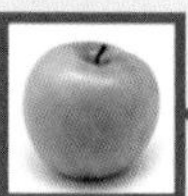

ORGANIZATIONS TO CONTACT

American Sleep Apnea Association (ASAA)

6856 Eastern Ave. NW, Ste. 203
Washington, DC 20012
Phone: (202) 293-3650
Fax: (202) 293-3656
E-mail: asaa@sleepapnea.org
Website: www.sleepapnea.org

The ASAA, founded in 1990, is a nonprofit organization that promotes awareness of sleep apnea and works for continuing improvements in treatments for this serious disease.

Centers for Disease Control and Prevention (CDC)

1600 Clifton Rd.
Atlanta, GA 30333
Phone: (800) 232-4636
Fax: (404) 235-1852
E-mail: cdcinfo@cdc.gov
Website: www.cdc.gov

The CDC's main mission is to protect the health of the American people by detecting and investigating health problems, including sleep disorders, and to conduct research to enhance prevention of those problems.

Narcolepsy Network

129 Waterwheel Ln.
North Kingstown, RI 02852
Phone: (888) 292-6522
Fax: (401) 633-6567
E-mail: narnet@narcolepsynetwork.org
Website: www.narcolepsynetwork.org

The Narcolepsy Network is a nonprofit organization dedicated to providing services to educate, advocate for, and support individuals with narcolepsy and related sleep disorders.

National Heart, Lung, and Blood Institute (NHLBI)

Bldg. 31, Rm. 5A52
31 Center Dr., MSC 2486
Bethesda, MD 20892
Phone: (301) 435-0199
Fax: (240) 629-3246
E-mail: nhlbiinfo@nhlbi.nih.gov
Website: www.nhlbi.nih.gov

The NHLBI provides global leadership for research, training, and education that promote the prevention and treatment of heart, lung, and blood diseases—including sleep disorders—and enhance the health of all those who suffer from them.

National Sleep Foundation (NSF)

1010 N. Glebe Rd., Ste. 310
Arlington, VA 22201
Phone: (703) 243-1697
E-mail: nsf@sleepfoundation.org
Website: www.sleepfoundation.org

The NSF's mission is to alert the public, health-care providers, and public-policy makers to the life-and-death importance of adequate sleep and to describe the symptoms and treatments of sleep disorders.

Restless Legs Syndrome Foundation

1530 Greenview Dr. SW, Ste. 210
Rochester, MN 55902
Phone: (507) 287-6465
Fax: (507) 287-6312
E-mail: rlsfoundation@rls.org
Website: www.rls.org

The Restless Legs Syndrome Foundation is a nonprofit organization that provides the latest information about RLS and works to increase awareness, improve treatments, and, through research, find a cure for RLS.

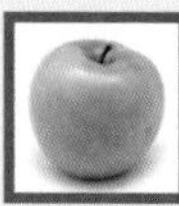

FOR MORE INFORMATION

Books

Faith H. Brynie. *101 Questions About Sleep and Dreams That Kept You Awake Nights . . . Until Now.* Minneapolis, MN: Twenty-First Century, 2006. This book contains useful information about teen sleeping habits, dreaming, what attending a sleep lab is like, and more.

L.H. Colligan. *Sleep Disorders.* New York: Marshall Cavendish, 2009. A general introduction to sleep problems, aimed at younger readers.

Judith P. Davidson. *Sink into Sleep: A Step-by-Step Guide for Reversing Insomnia.* New York: Demos Medical, 2013. A detailed but easy-to-read overview of insomnia and its possible cures.

Sylvia Engdahl. *Sleep Disorders.* Detroit: Greenhaven, 2011. A good general overview of sleep disorders, aimed at high school readers.

Lawrence J. Epstein. *The Harvard Medical School Guide to a Good Night's Sleep.* New York: McGraw-Hill, 2007. This well-written, authoritative book tells about the most common sleep disorders and how to avoid or cure them.

Max Hirshkowitz and Patricia B. Smith. *Sleep Disorders for Dummies.* Indianapolis, IN: Wiley, 2004. Do not be put off by the term *Dummies* in the title. This is a comprehensive, informative book cowritten by an internationally known authority on the subject.

Steven W. Lockely. *Sleep: A Very Short Introduction.* New York: Oxford University Press, 2012. In this easy-to-read book, the author discusses sleep through the ages, the reasons people need sleep, and how sleep affects human health.

Carlos H. Schenck. *Sleep.* New York: Avery, 2008. One of the country's leading sleep experts details the major sleep disorders, including their symptoms and how they are diagnosed and treated.

Barbara Sheen. *Sleep Disorders.* Detroit: Lucent, 2013. This well-written book explains the ins and outs of sleep disorders to young adult readers.

Internet Sources

American Psychological Association. "Why Sleep Is Important and What Happens When You Don't Get Enough." www.apa.org/topics/sleep/why.aspx?item=1.

Mayo Clinic staff. "Teen Sleep: Why Is Your Teen So Tired?" Mayo Clinic.

www.mayoclinic.com/health/teens-health/CC00019.

Restless Legs Syndrome Foundation. "About RLS." www.rls.org/page.aspx?pid=543#13.

Websites

How Sleeping Works, HowStuffWorks (http://science.howstuffworks.com/life/inside-the-mind/human-brain/sleep.htm). This large site, with several connected links, provides a convenient general overview of the basic facts about sleep, including brief but useful discussions of some of the major sleep disorders.

Sleep Terms, Definitions, and Abbreviations, Sleepnet.com (www.sleepnet.com/definition.html). A handy, detailed glossary of medical and other terms related to sleep and sleep disorders.

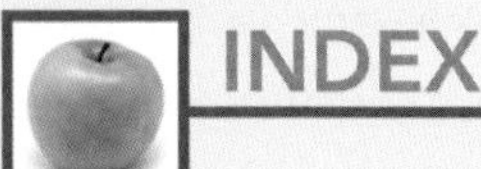

INDEX

P

R

S

T

V

PICTURE CREDITS

Cover: © Yuriy Rudyy/Shutterstock.com; © Brian Chase/Shutterstock.com; © Monkey Business Images/Shutterstock.com

© AgStock Images, Inc./Alamy, 10

© bikeriderlondon/Shutterstock.com, 13

© Bill Bachmann/Alamy, 42

© Bubbles Photolibrary/Alamy, 23, 55

© Catchlight Visual Services/Alamy, 17

© Chris Rout/Alamy, 25, 34, 78

© Chris Willson/Alamy, 40

© Donna E. Natale Planas/Miami Herald/MCT via Getty Images, 57

© Ernie James/Alamy, 21

© F1 ONLINE/SuperStock, 68

© Gale, Cengage, 16, 22

© Garo/Phanie/Science Source, 53

© Hank Morgan/Science Source, 14

© Ian Hooton/Science Source, 63

© Inga Spence/Science Source, 50

© J. Allan Hobson/Science Source, 81

© Janine Weidel Photolibrary/Alamy, 83

© Jim Zuckerman/Alamy, 37

© Joe Fox/Alamy, 75

© Mauro Fermariello/Science Source, 48

© Oleksiy Maksymenko Photography/Alamy, 31

© Patrick Kehoe/Alamy, 61

© Rob Marmion/Shutterstock.com, 77

© Science Source, 73

© Stephen Wood/Science Source, 71

© tab62/Shutterstock.com, 29

© Thierry Berrod, Mona Lisa Production/Science Source, 87

© Véronique Burger/Science Source, 45

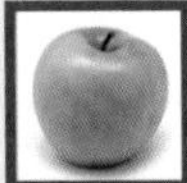

ABOUT THE AUTHOR

In addition to his numerous acclaimed volumes on ancient civilizations, historian Don Nardo has published several studies of modern scientific and medical discoveries and phenomena. Among these are *Germs*, *Atoms*, *Biological Warfare*, *Eating Disorders*, *Breast Cancer*, *Vaccines*, *Malnutrition*, *DNA Forensics*, and biographies of scientists Charles Darwin and Tycho Brahe. Nardo lives with his wife, Christine, in Massachusetts.